Stahl's Illustrated

Violence

Neural Circuits, Genetics and Treatment

Stephen M. Stahl
University of California, San Diego

Debbi Ann Morrissette
Neuroscience Education Institute

Nancy Muntner
Illustrations

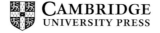

CAMBRIDGE
UNIVERSITY PRESS

CAMBRIDGE
UNIVERSITY PRESS

University Printing House, Cambridge CB2 8BS, United Kingdom

One Liberty Plaza, 20th Floor, New York, NY 10006, USA

477 Williamstown Road, Port Melbourne, VIC 3207, Australia

314-321, 3rd Floor, Plot 3, Splendor Forum, Jasola District Centre, New Delhi - 110025, India

79 Anson Road, #06-04/06, Singapore 079906

Cambridge University Press is part of the University of Cambridge.

It furthers the University's mission by disseminating knowledge in the pursuit of education, learning and research at the highest international levels of excellence.

www.cambridge.org
Information on this title: www.cambridge.org/9781107441606

© Neuroscience Education Institute 2014

First published 2014

A catalogue record for this publication is available from the British Library

ISBN 978-1-107-44160-6 Paperback

Cambridge University Press has no responsibility for the persistence or accuracy of URLs for external or third-party internet websites referred to in this publication, and does not guarantee that any content on such websites is, or will remain, accurate or appropriate.

....

Every effort has been made in preparing this book to provide accurate and up-to-date information which is in accord with accepted standards and practice at the time of publication. Although case histories are drawn from actual cases, every effort has been made to disguise the identities of the individuals involved. Nevertheless, the authors, editors and publishers can make no warranties that the information contained herein is totally free from error, not least because clinical standards are constantly changing through research and regulation. The authors, editors and publishers therefore disclaim all liability for direct or consequential damages resulting from the use of material contained in this book. Readers are strongly advised to pay careful attention to information provided by the manufacturer of any drugs or equipment that they plan to use.

PREFACE

This book is designed to be fun, with all concepts illustrated by full color images, figures, and tables supplemented by text. The visual learner will find that this book makes psychopharmacological concepts easier to master, and the non-visual learner may enjoy this book's short explanations of complex psychopharmacological concepts. Each chapter builds upon previous ones, synthesizing information about basic biology, diagnostics, treatment plans, complications, and comorbidities.

Novices may want to approach this book by first looking through all the graphics, gaining a feel for the visual vocabulary on which psychopharmacological concepts rely. After this once-over, we suggest going back through the book to read the text alongside the images. Learning from visual images and textual supplements should reinforce one another, providing novices with solid conceptual understanding at each step along the way.

Readers more familiar with these topics should find that going back and forth between the images and the text enables them to better understand complex psychopharmacological concepts. They may find themselves using this book frequently to refresh their psychopharmacological knowledge, and hopefully, they will refer their colleagues to this desk reference.

This book is intended as a conceptual overview of various topics. We provide you with a visual language to better understand the rules of psychopharmacology at the expense of discussing the exceptions to these rules. A Suggested Readings section at the back of this book gives you a good start for more in-depth learning about particular concepts.

Stahl's Essential Psychopharmacology (4th ed.) and *Stahl's Essential Psychopharmacology: The Prescriber's Guide* (4th ed.) can be helpful supplementary tools for more in-depth information on particular topics. You can also search the Neuroscience Education Institute's Web site (www.neiglobal.com) for articles, lectures, slides, and courses on psychopharmacological topics.

Whether you are a novice or an experienced psychopharmacologist, this book will hopefully lead you to think critically about the complexities of psychiatric disorders and their treatments.

Best wishes for your educational journey into the fascinating field of psychopharmacology!

Stephen M. Stahl

Table of Contents

CME Information

Overview
In this book, we will discuss what is known regarding individuals who are violent or aggressive, including neural circuitry and possible genetic influences underlying violent and aggressive behavior as well as the evidence- and practice-based treatment strategies that may reduce such behavior. Given the fact that mental illness may increase the risk of violent or aggressive behavior, yet with only a small subset of mentally ill patients exhibiting this disturbing behavior, it is crucial that we are able to predict which individuals are more likely to be violent or aggressive and take measures to prevent violent acts.

Target Audience
This activity has been developed for prescribers specializing in psychiatry. There are no prerequisites. All other health care providers interested in psychopharmacology are welcome for advanced study, especially primary care physicians, nurse practitioners, psychologists, and pharmacists.

Statement of Need
The following unmet needs and professional practice gaps regarding violence were revealed through new medical knowledge and following a critical analysis of activity feedback, expert faculty assessment, and a literature review:

- Increasingly, pressure is being put on mental health professionals to better predict which individuals are at the greatest risk for committing acts of violence

- There is also great demand for clinicians to employ treatment strategies aimed at preventing violent and aggressive behavior

- There is little evidence-based psychopharmacology for the management of treatment-resistant aggressive symptoms in individuals with violence and assaultiveness other than clozapine

- Standard doses of all antipsychotics target 60-80% occupancy of D2 receptors, but this may principally treat positive symptoms and be effective only in individuals who are neither treatment resistant nor violent; very high-dose antipsychotic treatment to target >80% D2 receptor occupancy may be justified in individual cases

To help address clinician performance gaps with respect to understanding and treating violent or aggressive behavior, quality improvement efforts need to provide education regarding 1) the epidemiology, neurobiology, and genetics of violence, impulsivity, and aggression and 2) strategies to address violent, impulsive, and aggressive behavior in patients with mental illness.

Learning Objectives
After completing this activity, participants should be better able to:

- Understand the epidemiology and heterogeneity of violence and aggression
- Utilize knowledge of environmental and genetic risk factors for predicting which individuals may become violent or aggressive
- Explore the neurobiological factors thought to underlie violent and aggressive behavior
- Apply evidence-based treatment strategies to individuals with violent or aggressive behavior

Accreditation and Credit Designation Statements
The Neuroscience Education Institute is accredited by the Accreditation Council for Continuing Medical Education (ACCME) to provide continuing medical education for physicians.

The Neuroscience Education Institute designates this enduring material for a maximum of 6.0 *AMA PRA Category 1 Credits*™. Physicians should claim only the credit commensurate with the extent of their participation in the activity.

Nurses: for all of your CNE requirements for recertification, the ANCC will accept *AMA PRA Category 1 Credits*™ from organizations accredited by the ACCME.

Physician Assistants: the NCCPA accepts *AMA PRA Category 1 Credits*™ from organizations accredited by the AMA (providers accredited by the ACCME).

A certificate of participation for completing this activity is available.

Activity Instructions
This CME activity is in the form of a printed monograph and incorporates instructional design to enhance your retention of the information presented. You are advised to go through the figures in this activity from beginning to end, followed by the text, and then complete the posttest and activity evaluation. The estimated time for completion of this activity is 6.0 hours.

Instructions for CME Credit
To receive your certificate of CME credit or participation, please complete the posttest and evaluation, available only online at **www.neiglobal.com/CME** (under "Book"). If a passing score of 70% or more is attained (required to receive credit), you can immediately print your certificate. There is a fee for the posttest for this

activity (waived for NEI members). If you have questions, please call 888-535-5600 or email customerservice@neiglobal.com.

NEI Disclosure Policy
It is the policy of the Neuroscience Education Institute to ensure balance, independence, objectivity, and scientific rigor in all its educational activities. Therefore, all individuals in a position to influence or control content development are required by NEI to disclose any financial relationships or apparent conflicts of interest. Although potential conflicts of interest are identified and resolved prior to the activity, it remains for the audience to determine whether outside interests reflect a possible bias in either the exposition or the conclusions presented.

These materials have been peer reviewed to ensure the scientific accuracy and medical relevance of the information presented and its independence from commercial bias. The Neuroscience Education Institute takes responsibility for the content, quality, and scientific integrity of this CME activity.

Individual Disclosure Statements
Authors/Developers
Debbi Ann Morrissette, PhD
Adjunct Professor, Biological Sciences, California State University, San Marcos, CA
Adjunct Professor, Biological Sciences, Palomar Community College, San Marcos, CA
Senior Medical Writer, Neuroscience Education Institute, Carlsbad, CA
No financial relationships to disclose

Stephen M. Stahl, MD, PhD
Adjunct Professor, Department of Psychiatry, University of California, San Diego School of Medicine
Honorary Visiting Senior Fellow, University of Cambridge, UK
Director of Psychopharmacology, California Department of State Hospitals
Grant/Research: Avanir, CeNeRx, Forest, Genomind, Lilly, Janssen, Mylan, Otsuka America, Pamlab, Servier, Shire, Sunovion, Takeda
Consultant/Advisor: Avanir, BioMarin, Depomed, Forest, Genentech, Genomind, GlaxoSmithKline, Jazz, Merck, Navigant, Novartis, Noveida, Neuronetics, Orexigen, Otsuka America, Pamlab, Reviva, Roche, Shire, Sunovion, Taisho, Teva, Trius
Speakers Bureau: Arbor Scientia, Genomind, Janssen, Lilly, Pamlab, Pfizer, Sunovion, Takeda
Board Member: Genomind, RCT Logic

Peer Reviewer
Steven S. Simring, MD, MPH
Clinical Associate Professor, Department of Psychiatry, Columbia University College of Physicians and Surgeons, New York State Psychiatric Institute, New York City
No financial relationships to disclose

Design Staff
Nancy Muntner, *Director, Medical Illustrations, Neuroscience Education Institute, Carlsbad, CA*
No financial relationships to disclose

Program Development
Steve Smith, *President and CEO, Neuroscience Education Institute, Carlsbad, CA*
No financial relationships to disclose

Disclosed financial relationships with conflicts of interest have been reviewed by the Neuroscience Education Institute CME Advisory Board Chair and resolved. All faculty and planning committee members have attested that their financial relationships, if any, do not affect their ability to present well-balanced, evidence-based content for this activity.

Disclosure of Off-Label Use
This educational activity may include discussion of unlabeled and/or investigational uses of agents that are not currently labeled for such use by the FDA. Please consult the product prescribing information for full disclosure of labeled uses.

Disclaimer
Participants have an implied responsibility to use the newly acquired information from this activity to enhance patient outcomes and their own professional development. The information presented in this educational activity is not meant to serve as a guideline for patient management. Any procedures, medications, or other courses of diagnosis or treatment discussed or suggested in this educational activity should not be used by clinicians without evaluation of their patients' conditions and possible contraindications or dangers in use, review of any applicable manufacturer's product information, and comparison with recommendations from other authorities. Primary references and full prescribing information should be consulted.

Sponsorship Information
This activity is sponsored by the Neuroscience Education Institute.

Support
This activity is supported solely by the sponsor, Neuroscience Education Institute.

Date of Release/Expiration
Released: March 1, 2014
CME credit expires: February 28, 2017. *If this date has passed, please contact NEI for updated information.*

Stahl's Illustrated | Objectives

- Describe the epidemiology and heterogeneity of violence and aggression

- Utilize knowledge of environmental and genetic risk factors to predict which individuals may become violent or aggressive

- Explore the neurobiological factors thought to underlie violent and aggressive behavior

- Apply evidence-based assessment and treatment strategies to individuals with violent or aggressive behavior

Introduction

Increasingly, pressure is being put on mental health professionals to better predict which individuals are at the greatest risk of committing acts of violence. There is also great demand for clinicians to employ treatment strategies aimed at preventing violent and aggressive behavior. In this book, we will discuss what is known about violent and aggressive individuals, including neural circuitry and possible genetic influences underlying violent and aggressive behavior as well as evidence- and practice-based treatment strategies that may reduce such behavior. Given the fact that mental illness may increase the risk of violent or aggressive behavior, yet with only a small subset of mentally ill patients exhibiting this disturbing behavior, it is crucial to be able to predict which individuals are more likely to be violent or aggressive and take measures to prevent violent acts.

Which Individuals Will Become Violent or Aggressive?

Chapter 1 discusses the different types of aggressive behavior (impulsive, psychotic, and psychopathic), each likely with unique neurobiological substrates. Various risk factors for violence and aggression, especially in mental illness, are also described. These risk factors include childhood maltreatment, substance abuse, cognitive dysfunction, and treatment nonadherence. In conjunction with several available violence risk assessment tools, clinical evaluation of known risk factors should aid clinicians in determining which individuals are most likely to become violent or aggressive.

The Heterogeneity of Violence

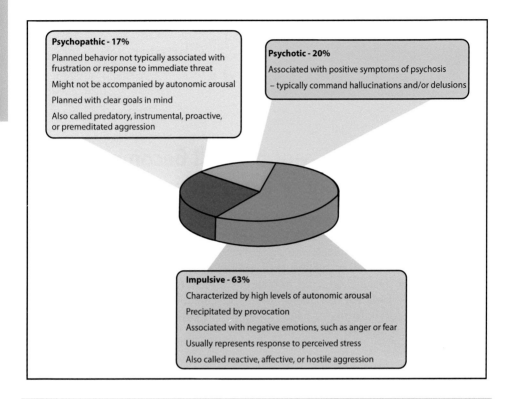

Psychopathic - 17%

Planned behavior not typically associated with frustration or response to immediate threat

Might not be accompanied by autonomic arousal

Planned with clear goals in mind

Also called predatory, instrumental, proactive, or premeditated aggression

Psychotic - 20%

Associated with positive symptoms of psychosis

– typically command hallucinations and/or delusions

Impulsive - 63%

Characterized by high levels of autonomic arousal

Precipitated by provocation

Associated with negative emotions, such as anger or fear

Usually represents response to perceived stress

Also called reactive, affective, or hostile aggression

FIGURE 1.1. Aggression can be defined as hostile, injurious, or destructive behavior that may have various targets (self- or other-directed) and different modes of action (physical or verbal, direct or indirect). There are at least 3 different types of aggression, including psychotic, impulsive, and psychopathic. Approximately 20% of violent acts are of the psychotic variety; the majority of the rest are due to lack of impulse control (Nolan et al., 2003). Only a relatively small portion of violent acts are due to psychopathy; however, this type of violence seems to be the most lethal and the least responsive to treatment (Citrome and Volavka, 2011; Swanson et al., 2008; Volavka and Citrome, 2008). Each of these types of aggression may be attributable to dysfunction in distinct neural circuits. Identifying the type of aggression a patient is displaying may help guide the selection of appropriate treatments that target the underlying dysfunctional circuits. However, violence and aggression arise from a complex combination of neurobiological, genetic, and environmental factors and are often presented in the context of comorbid conditions. Thus, the assessment and treatment of violence and aggression can be quite complicated.

Impulsive Aggression

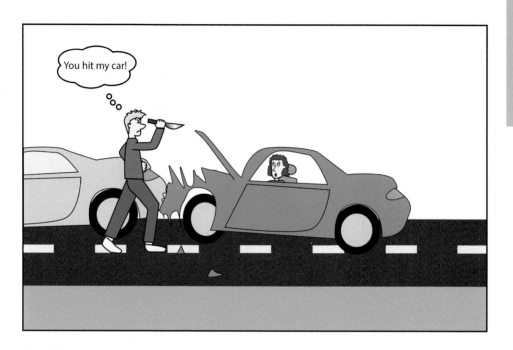

FIGURE 1.2. Impulsive, or reactive, aggression involves no planning and is usually an immediate response to an environmental stimulus. Impulsive aggression may reflect emotional hypersensitivity and exaggerated threat perception.

Psychotic Aggression

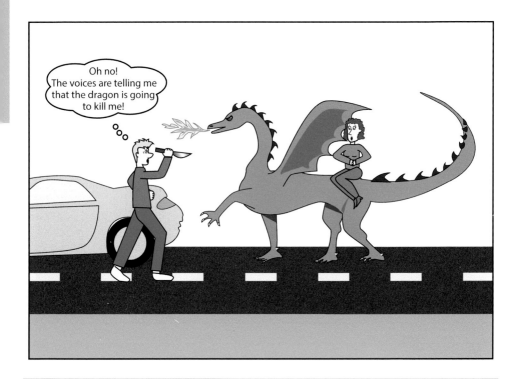

FIGURE 1.3. Psychotic violence is attributable to positive symptoms of psychosis, most commonly paranoid delusions of threat or persecution, command hallucinations, and grandiosity. Such psychotic symptoms may lead to violent behavior due to the assailant misunderstanding or misinterpreting environmental stimuli. In line with this, a recent study determined that 59% of individuals with schizophrenia who had committed acts of homicide were experiencing delusions, with a worsening of delusions in the months leading up to the homicidal act.

Psychopathic Aggression

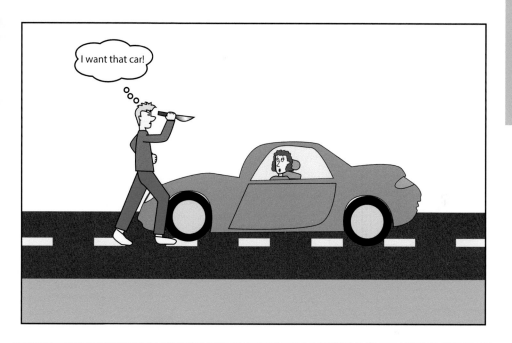

FIGURE 1.4. Psychopathic violence involves aggressive acts characterized by the planning of assaults, predatory gain, and lack of remorse.

Risk Factors for Violent Behavior

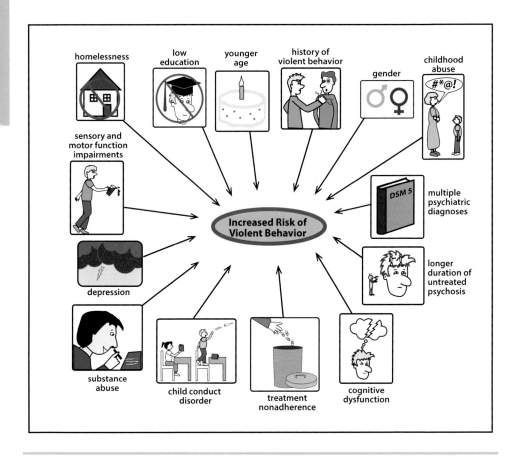

FIGURE 1.5. Several factors have been associated with a risk of violent or aggressive behavior, including a history of prior violence, childhood conduct disorder, childhood abuse or trauma, substance abuse, low education, younger age (under 25 years), homelessness, sensory and motor function impairments, cognitive dysfunction, including poor illness insight, low treatment satisfaction, longer duration of untreated psychosis, treatment nonadherence, depression, multiple psychiatric diagnoses, and possibly gender.

Child Abuse as a Risk Factor for Violent Behavior

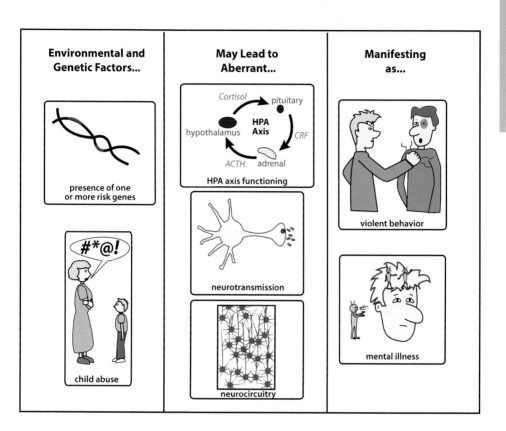

| Environmental and Genetic Factors... | May Lead to Aberrant... | Manifesting as... |

presence of one or more risk genes

HPA axis functioning

neurotransmission

neurocircuitry

child abuse

violent behavior

mental illness

FIGURE 1.6. Childhood abuse or neglect has been linked to an increased risk of delinquency and violent criminal behavior as well as measures of lifetime aggression. Maltreatment at a young age may have detrimental effects on the developing brain, leading to aberrant neural circuitry and maladaptive neurotransmitter release. Data also indicate that highly aggressive behavior is correlated with low cortisol levels. Interestingly, childhood trauma may cause dysfunction in stress response behavior by altering stress hormone (e.g., cortisol) levels and impairing hypothalamic-pituitary-adrenal (HPA) axis functioning. Individuals who are at an increased biological risk of the development of mental illness due to genetic factors may be particularly vulnerable to the detrimental effects of adverse psychosocial experiences.

Substance Abuse as a Risk Factor for Violent Behavior

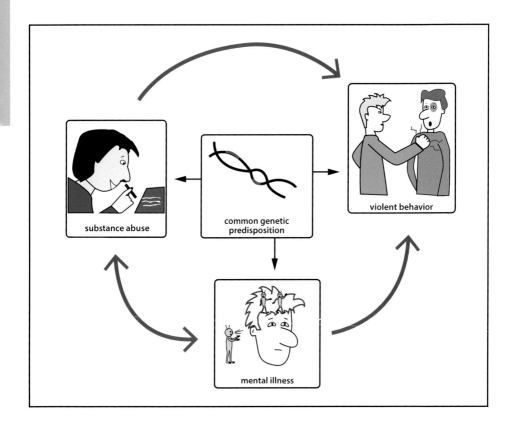

FIGURE 1.7. Substance use disorder (SUD) in and of itself confers an increased risk of violence. SUD is highly prevalent in patients with mental illness; however, the exact relationship between SUD, mental illness, and aggression is not fully understood (Fazel et al., 2009a; Fazel et al., 2009c). It is possible that mental illnesses such as schizophrenia and bipolar disorder predispose individuals to the development of SUD as well as violent or aggressive behavior. It is also possible that SUD increases the risk of developing a psychiatric disorder and exhibiting violent or aggressive behavior. Furthermore, substances of abuse may lead to violent or aggressive acts due to their disinhibitory effects on impulse control. It is also possible that there is a common genetic susceptibility underlying certain psychiatric disorders, SUD, and aggressive behavior. Regardless of the exact mechanism underlying the correlation between mental illness, SUD, and violence, it is clear that addressing substance abuse may help prevent acts of violence and aggression.

Schizophrenia May Increase the Risk of Violent Behavior

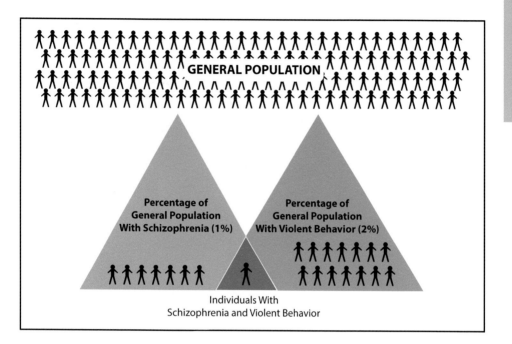

GENERAL POPULATION

Percentage of General Population With Schizophrenia (1%)

Percentage of General Population With Violent Behavior (2%)

Individuals With Schizophrenia and Violent Behavior

FIGURE 1.8. Although not all patients with mental illness are violent or aggressive, there is a small subset of the mentally ill population who are at a higher risk of violent behavior than the general population. In fact, patients with schizophrenia are at a 4–6-fold increased risk of exhibiting violent or aggressive behavior. As many as 10% of individuals with a psychotic disorder are violent; in comparison, only 2% of individuals in the general population display such behavior (Fazel and Grann, 2006; Fazel et al., 2009a; Fazel et al., 2009b). This prevalence value may actually be underestimated, as one recent study indicated that within a 6-month time frame, as many as 50% of patients with schizophrenia had committed an act of violence (Fazel et al., 2009a). In terms of severely violent behavior (e.g., homicide), individuals with psychosis may be as high as 20 times more likely than the general population to commit acts of severe violence. However, only 5.2% of severely violent crimes are committed by individuals with a psychiatric disorder, most commonly schizophrenia (Fazel and Grann, 2006). Thus, although we strive to avoid the misconception that all patients with schizophrenia are violent, the data indicate that schizophrenia, especially when untreated, significantly increases the risk of displaying violent behavior. It should be emphasized that violence occurs not because of a diagnosis of schizophrenia in and of itself; rather, violence is often associated with acute psychotic states.

The Cost of Violence in Schizophrenia

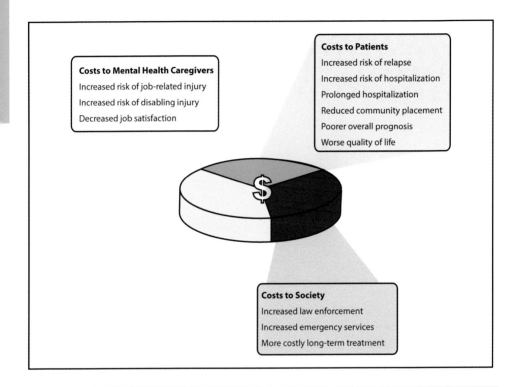

Costs to Mental Health Caregivers
Increased risk of job-related injury
Increased risk of disabling injury
Decreased job satisfaction

Costs to Patients
Increased risk of relapse
Increased risk of hospitalization
Prolonged hospitalization
Reduced community placement
Poorer overall prognosis
Worse quality of life

Costs to Society
Increased law enforcement
Increased emergency services
More costly long-term treatment

FIGURE 1.9. Violent behavior in patients with schizophrenia has several costs to patients, mental health caregivers, and society. For the patient, violent behavior has been shown to prolong inpatient duration and inhibit community placement. In general, violent behavior is also associated with a poorer prognosis. Mental health caregivers may be at a greater risk of experiencing job-related violent crime than workers in many other occupations (Anderson and West, 2011). In fact, approximately 25% of psychiatric nurses may be the victim of a patient assault that results in disabling injury (Quanbeck et al., 2007).

Gender as a Risk Factor
for Violent Behavior

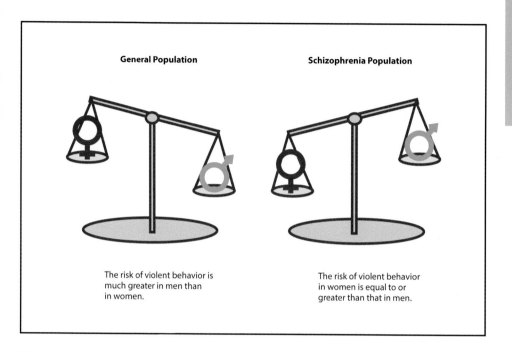

General Population

Schizophrenia Population

The risk of violent behavior is much greater in men than in women.

The risk of violent behavior in women is equal to or greater than that in men.

FIGURE 1.10. Although men in the general population are at a greater risk of demonstrating violent or aggressive behavior, in the schizophrenia population, women are at an equal or even greater risk of such behavior (Dean et al., 2006; Taylor and Bragado-Jimenez, 2009). Interestingly, despite the increased incidence of violence in female compared to male psychiatric patients, clinicians may be much less successful in predicting violent behavior in female patients (Lids et al., 1993).

"Sexual Unmorphism" in Schizophrenia

Sexual "Unmorphism" in Schizophrenia	
Normal Sexual Dimorphism	**Reversal in Schizophrenia**
Male brains are more lateralized	Reduced lateralization in males with schizophrenia
Females have a smaller hypothalamus	Females with schizophrenia have a larger hypothalamus than healthy females
Females have greater gray matter volume in the anterior cingulate cortex	Reduced anterior cingulate volume in females with schizophrenia
Females display less aggression than males	Females with schizophrenia are more aggressive than healthy females
Females have a greater orbitofrontal cortex:amygdala ratio (OAR)	Males with schizophrenia have a higher OAR than healthy males
	Females with schizophrenia have a smaller OAR than healthy females
The pattern of brain activation during emotional processing is sexually dimorphic	Males with schizophrenia exhibit a pattern of brain activation more similar to that of healthy females
	Females with schizophrenia exhibit a pattern of brain activation more similar to that of healthy males

More feminine   *More masculine*   *Sexually dimorphic*

FIGURE 1.11. Sexual dimorphism of the human brain, whereby brain structure and connectivity varies between the sexes, has long been recognized. However, this sexual dimorphism is altered in schizophrenia, with female patients demonstrating more masculine features and vice versa. Indeed, at the neurobiological level, structures that are typically larger in healthy male brains, including the hypothalamus, are of equal size in or are reversed between men and women with schizophrenia. Likewise, structures that are typically larger in the healthy female brain, including the anterior cingulate cortex, are of equal size in or are reversed between men and women with schizophrenia (Holden, 2005). Women with schizophrenia also process certain information in a more male-typical manner, while men with schizophrenia tend to use more female-typical processing schemas (Guillem et al., 2009; Mendrek and Stip, 2011).

Testosterone Exposure and Schizophrenia

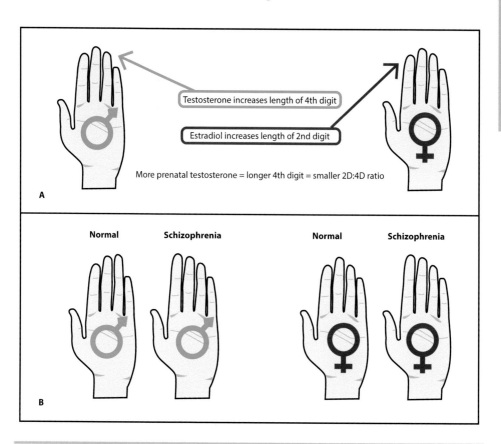

FIGURE 1.12. One possible connection between the reversal of sexual dimorphism, or "sexual unmorphism," in schizophrenia may depend on the role of testosterone levels both during development and throughout the lifespan. A) A fascinating body of research has determined that hormone exposure in utero may be evidenced by digit length, whereby testosterone levels increase the length of the fourth digit (the ring finger) and estradiol increases the length of the second digit (the pointer finger) (Manning et al., 1998; McIntyre, 2006). B) In adult patients with schizophrenia, the ratio between the lengths of the second and fourth digits is altered, indicating exposure to elevated estradiol or decreased testosterone in utero (Arato et al., 2004). This phenomena is especially interesting given that maternal stress, which decreases testosterone levels, has been associated with an increased risk of schizophrenia in men (Morgan and Bale, 2011).

Testosterone and Violent Behavior

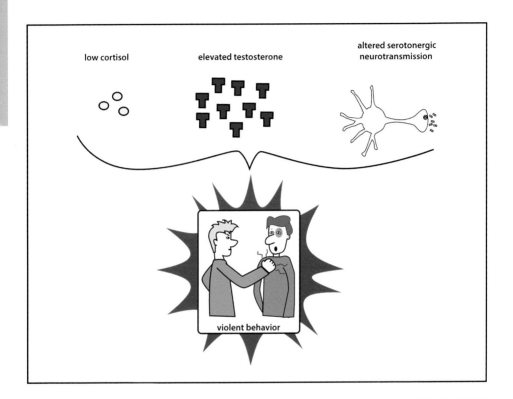

FIGURE 1.13. Increased testosterone levels in healthy adults have traditionally been positively correlated with increased aggressive behavior, although not all studies support this idea. More recent evidence suggests that elevated testosterone levels alone do not predict aggressive behavior; a concomitant decrease in cortisol and perhaps altered serotonergic neurotransmission must also be present to accurately predict aggressive behavior.

Testosterone, Serotonin, and Impulsive Aggression

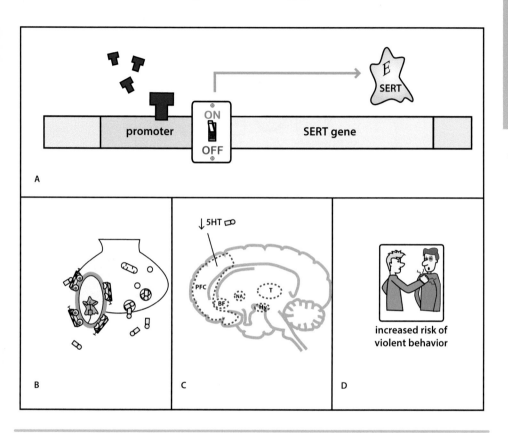

FIGURE 1.14. Interestingly, impulsive aggression in men has been associated with high testosterone concentration coupled with low serotonergic activity, possibly due to the upregulation of serotonin transporter (SERT) mRNA by testosterone. A) The binding of testosterone to the promoter region of the SERT gene may increase the production of SERT. B) SERT is the transporter responsible for the reuptake of serotonin (5HT) from the synapse, leading to C) reduced 5HT levels, especially in the prefrontal cortex (PFC). D) The combination of elevated testosterone and decreased 5HT may increase the risk of impulsive aggression. This reduction in serotonergic activity observed in impulsively aggressive individuals is not found in patients with psychopathic aggression, further supporting the heterogeneous nature of violent behavior (Comai et al., 2012a).

Testosterone, Cognition, and Hostility in Patients With Schizophrenia

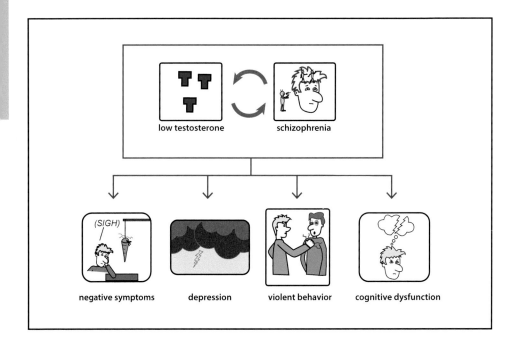

FIGURE 1.15. Somewhat counterintuitively, male patients with schizophrenia tend to have lower levels of testosterone despite being at an increased risk of violent or aggressive behavior. Testosterone might be lower in patients with schizophrenia as a result of the disorder itself, and/or it may be that low testosterone during neurodevelopment contributes to the development of schizophrenia. Performance on various cognitive tasks, including verbal and working memory tests, is correlated with low testosterone levels in patients with schizophrenia but not in healthy male control subjects. In patients with schizophrenia, low testosterone is also correlated with increased hostility as well as increased negative symptoms of schizophrenia (Moore et al., 2013).

Testosterone Modulates Cortical and Subcortical Neurocircuitry

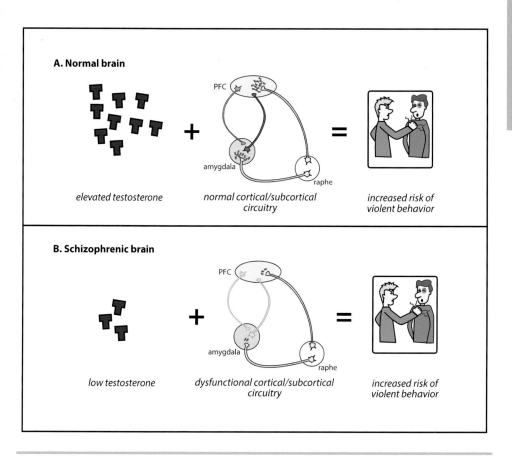

FIGURE 1.16. Recent data indicate that endogenous testosterone modulates serotonergic neurotransmission as well as connectivity between the PFC and the amygdala in healthy men (Volman et al., 2011). Both of these brain regions as well as the serotonergic system are implicated in the neurobiology of aggression and may be dysfunctional in schizophrenia as well as psychopathy. Therefore, the apparent discrepancy between testosterone being A) positively correlated with aggression in healthy men and B) negatively correlated with aggression in male patients with schizophrenia may be a product of testosterone acting on dysfunctional cortical and subcortical circuitry in the schizophrenic brain.

Cognitive Dysfunction as a Risk Factor for Violent Behavior

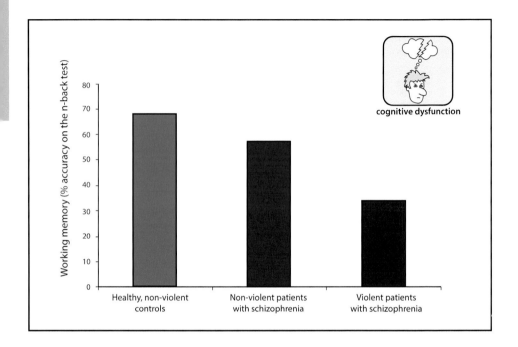

FIGURE 1.17. Along with positive, negative, and affective symptom domains, cognitive dysfunction is a prominent feature of schizophrenia. Not all patients with schizophrenia and cognitive deficits exhibit aggressive behavior; however, several studies have indicated that violent patients with schizophrenia have greater cognitive dysfunction than non-violent patients with schizophrenia (Singh et al., 2011b; Song and Min, 2009). Cognitive dysfunction, especially deficits in executive function, may increase the risk of violence in schizophrenia because patients lack the ability to cognitively suppress impulsive drives coming from limbic areas or learn from the consequences of violent actions. Some recently published studies indicate that improvement in cognitive dysfunction correlates with improvement in aggressive behavior (Krakowski and Czobor, 2012; Krakowski et al., 2008).

Affective Disorder as a
Risk Factor for Violent Behavior

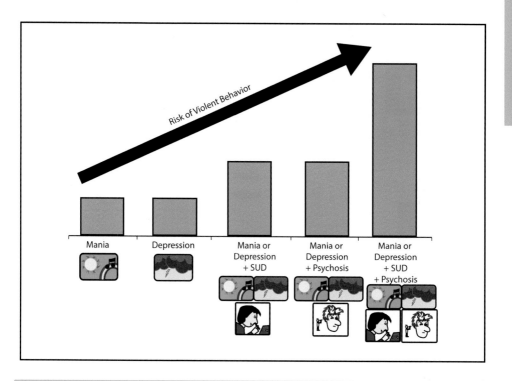

FIGURE 1.18. Individuals with an affective disorder, in particular bipolar disorder, are associated with a higher risk of violent or aggressive behavior than the general population. This increased risk is greater in individuals currently having a mood episode but seems to be independent of type of episode (depressive, manic, hypomanic, or mixed). The correlation between bipolar disorder and violent behavior may be strongest when comorbid psychosis or SUD is also present.

Treatment Nonadherence as a
Risk Factor for Violent Behavior

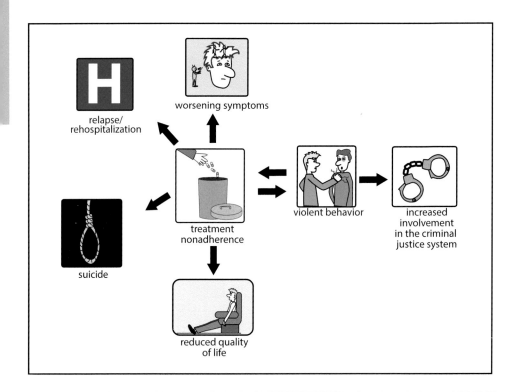

FIGURE 1.19. Treatment nonadherence has been associated with several adverse outcomes in schizophrenia, including symptom worsening, suicide, increased relapse and rehospitalization, and reduced satisfaction with life. Gaps in therapy of even 1–10 days double the likelihood of rehospitalization (Weiden et al., 2004). Additionally, treatment nonadherence in schizophrenia may increase the risk of violent or aggressive behavior. One recent study indicated that involvement in the criminal justice system may be yet another consequence of treatment nonadherence in patients with schizophrenia (Ascher-Svanum et al., 2010). Conversely, rising hostility may predict the development of treatment nonadherence in patients with schizophrenia. However, it is important to note that treatment adherence does not preclude violence in patients with schizophrenia; even patients who are adherent to medication may exhibit violent or aggressive behavior (Bobes et al., 2009). The association between treatment nonadherence and violence in schizophrenia may be at least partially attributable to the need for high, continued occupancy of dopamine D2 receptors in some patients.

Violence Risk Assessment Tools

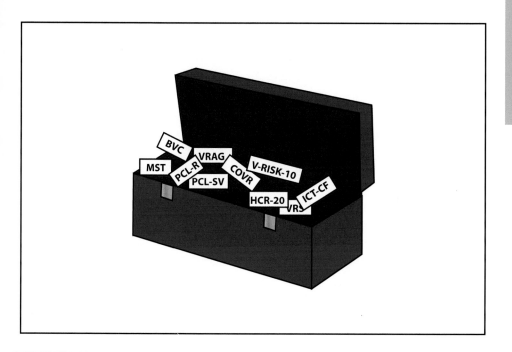

FIGURE 1.20. There are several tools available that may help clinicians predict which of their patients may become violent and thus take measures to prevent acts of violence. These tools include the Historical Clinical Risk Management (HCR-20), the Hare Psychopathy Checklist-Revised (PCL-R), the Hare Psychopathy Checklist: Screening Version (PCL:SV), the Brøset Violence Checklist (BVC), the Classification of Violence Risk (COVR), the Violence Risk Assessment Guide (VRAG), the Violence Risk Screening-10 (V-RISK-10), the Violence Risk Scale (VRS), the Clinically Feasible Iterative Classification Tree (ICT-CF), and the Modified Screening Tool (MST). However, as few as 10% of mental health professionals may actually utilize such assessment tools and instead rely on clinical judgment.

Violence Risk Assessment: Patient Prediction

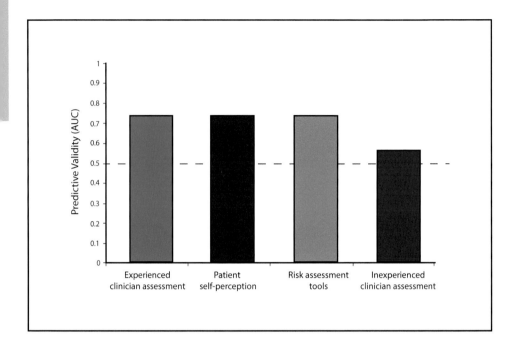

FIGURE 1.21. Although assessment tools have their limitations, clinical judgment may be even less accurate, especially for mental health professionals with limited clinical experience. Perhaps surprisingly, a recent study suggests that accurate predictions of future violence may come from patients themselves (Skeem et al., 2013). Patients were asked a single question regarding the probability that they would commit a violent or aggressive act in the next 2 months. Patient self-perception of violence risk strongly correlated with actual incidence of violent acts. This study specifically excluded patients with a diagnosis of schizophrenia, so it is not yet known if these results apply to that particular population. It is likely that a risk assessment that utilizes a combination of available screening tools, clinical judgment, and perhaps patient self-perception may be best for predicting the probability that a patient will commit a future act of violence.

Chapter 2

Neurobiology and Genetics of Violence and Aggression

Violent behavior is thought to be associated with dysfunction in various neurotransmitter systems in both the prefrontal cortical and limbic areas. Dysfunction in these systems seems to be impacted by many different genetic polymorphisms, but it is also heavily reliant upon adverse experiences during development as well as gender. By understanding which circuits, genes, and systems underlie aggression and violence, the astute clinician will be better prepared to understand why an individual may become violent or aggressive.

Neural Circuits Involved in Aggressive Behavior

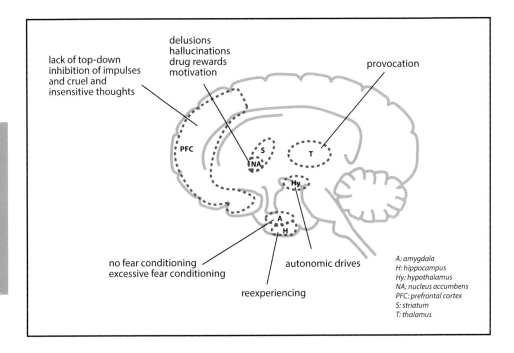

FIGURE 2.1. Impaired neurotransmission in various brain regions may contribute to the propensity for violent or aggressive behavior. The specific type of aggressive behavior is likely correlated with dysfunction in specific neural circuits. For example, both impulsive and psychotic aggression have been hypothesized to involve excessive reactivity to perceived threats (bottom-up out of control) and inadequate cortical regulation (top-down out of control). Although they are perhaps present in all patients with schizophrenia, structural and functional abnormalities in the frontal and temporal cortices as well as reduced connectivity between these brain areas may be more severe in aggressive patients than in those who are not aggressive. In the amygdala, fear conditioning seems to be excessive in both psychotic and impulsive aggression, whereas individuals with psychopathic aggression seem to lack fear conditioning.

Bottom-Up Drive and Top-Down Brake

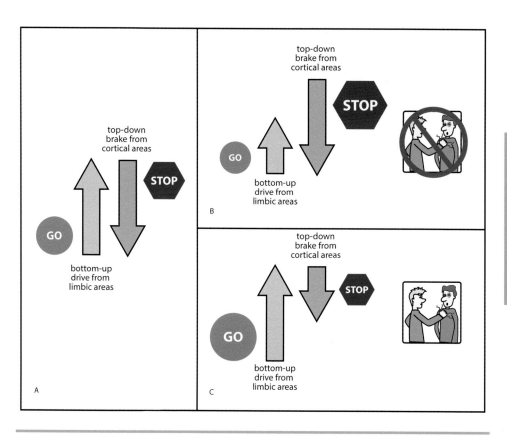

FIGURE 2.2. A) Impulsive drives in response to perceived threats stem from limbic regions, including the amygdala. Activity in limbic regions is modulated by input from cortical brain regions, including the prefrontal cortex (PFC). The balance between this limbic drive and the opposing cortical brakes determines whether one will act out an impulsive behavior such as aggression. B) If the limbic drive is not overly strong, and/or if the cortical brake is sufficient to control impulsive drives coming from limbic areas, an individual will not act out with violent or aggressive behavior. C) If the limbic drive is overly strong, and/or if the cortical brake system is not strong enough, an individual will be at an increased risk of violent behavior.

Top-Down Cortical Control

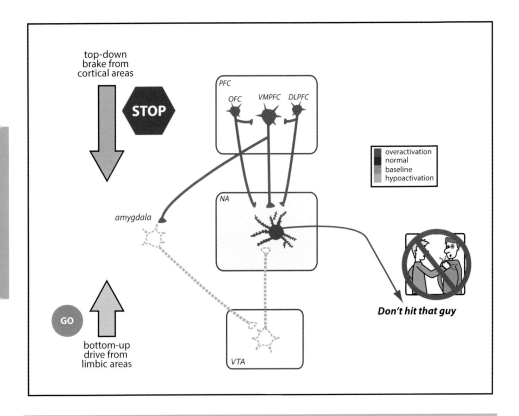

FIGURE 2.3. Top-down control is most strongly associated with portions of the PFC, including the dorsolateral PFC (DLPFC), the ventromedial PFC (VMPFC), and the orbitofrontal cortex (OFC). These regions are involved in decision making, and dysfunction in these areas results in a lack of recognition of consequences, the inability to use previously learned information about reward and punishment, the misinterpretation of emotionally neutral stimuli as negative, and impaired recognition of social cues. VTA: ventral tegmental area

Bottom-Up Limbic Control

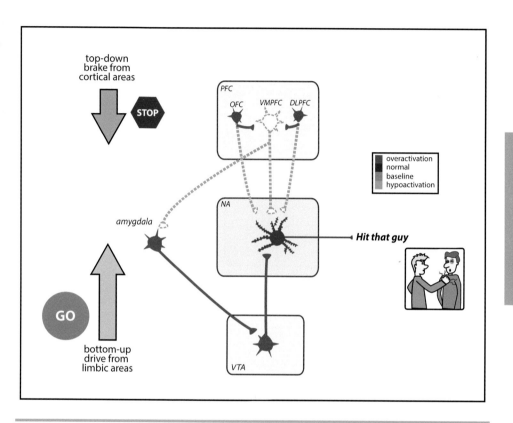

FIGURE 2.4. The amygdala is involved in the rapid detection of threat as well as the excitation of fight-or-flight responses. The amygdala is hyperactive in impulsive aggression but hypoactive in psychopathic aggression. Aggressive behavior may also stem from abnormalities in other limbic regions, including the anterior cingulate cortex (ACC), the hippocampus, the thalamus, and the hypothalamus. The thalamus is involved in the filtering of incoming information, whereas the ACC is thought to be involved in the organization and relaying of information; dysfunction in these brain regions may lead to overstimulation that results in impulsive behavior. Indeed, violent individuals with schizophrenia show decreased thalamic activation and larger caudate nucleus volume compared to nonviolent individuals with schizophrenia (Barkataki et al., 2008).

Neurocircuitry of Impulsive Aggression

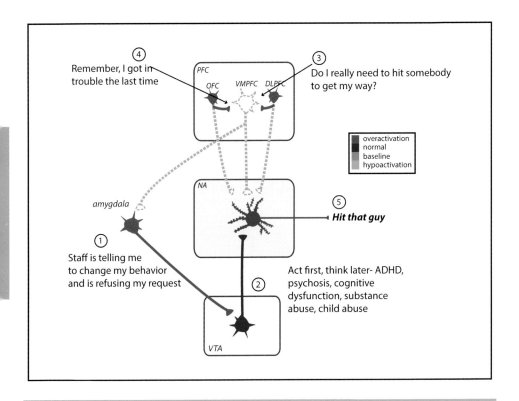

FIGURE 2.5. Impulsive aggression, such as that which occurs in attention deficit hyperactivity disorder (ADHD), posttraumatic stress disorder (PTSD), substance use disorder (SUD), and borderline personality disorder, is likely due in part to impaired cortical control, often coupled with excessive limbic drive (Coccaro et al., 2007; Coccaro et al., 2011; De Sanctis et al., 2012). 1) The amygdala is disproportionately hyperactivated in response to a perceived environmental stressor or threat. 2) Input from the amygdala to the ventral tegmental area (VTA) and from the VTA to the nucleus accumbens (NA) is a driving force compelling the individual to act out in a violent or aggressive manner. In individuals prone to impulsive aggression, the usual top-down cortical brakes are insufficient to counterbalance the limbic drive. This cortical input normally allows healthy individuals to 3) evaluate the situation rationally, 4) consider the consequences of aggressive action, and 5) suppress the behavior. Those with disorders associated with impulsive violence often cannot do these things.

Neurocircuitry of
Psychotic Aggression

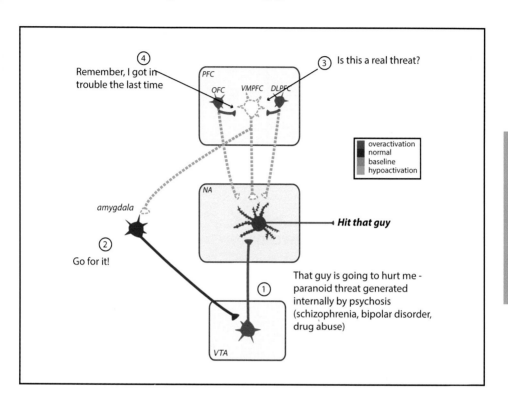

FIGURE 2.6. In psychotic aggression, 1) the initial drive likely comes from striatal hyperactivity due to psychosis, such as that which occurs in schizophrenia, bipolar disorder, and substance abuse. When coupled with 2) normal limbic drive and insufficient cortical input due to impairment in 3) the DLPFC as well as 4) the OFC and the VMPFC, an individual with a psychotic illness may act out with violence or aggression in response to a perceived threat.

Psychopathy Defined

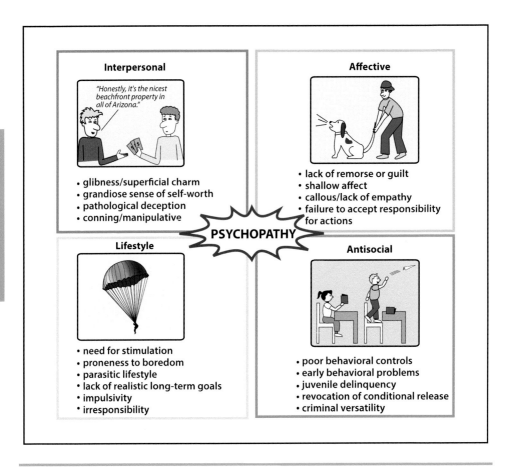

FIGURE 2.7. Psychopathic (also called predatory, instrumental, or proactive) aggression manifests as planned behavior not typically associated with frustration or response to an immediate threat; in fact, there is often no accompanying autonomic arousal. According to the Psychopathology Checklist–Revised (PCL-R), the assessment of psychopathology is based on ratings in 4 dimensions: interpersonal, affective, lifestyle, and antisocial. A score of 30 or more indicates that an individual has psychopathy (Hare and Neumann, 2008).

Conduct Disorder, ASPD, and Psychopathy

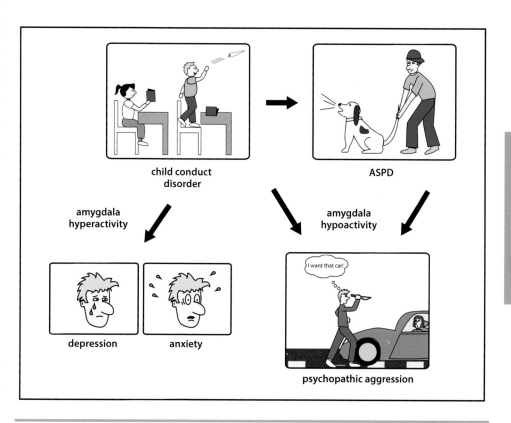

FIGURE 2.8. While most individuals with psychopathy demonstrate conduct disorder as children as well as antisocial personality disorder (ASPD), not all individuals with conduct disorder or ASPD have features of psychopathy (Kosson et al., 2006). Conduct disorder is a childhood disorder with persistent aggressive or antisocial behavior, whereas APSD describes individuals who chronically engage in irresponsible and criminal behavior (Glenn et al., 2013; Blair, 2013). Individuals with ASPD and psychopathy are much more likely to commit violent acts (Kosson et al., 2006). Interestingly, one recent study found that among individuals with schizophrenia and a history of crime, 67% had a history of childhood conduct disorder, 73% had comorbid ASPD, and 40% had comorbid psychopathy (versus 30% with conduct disorder, 10% with ASPD, and 0% with psychopathy among individuals with schizophrenia and no criminal history) (Maghsoodloo et al., 2012). These data underscore the complex nature of violent behavior.

Neurocircuitry of Psychopathic Aggression

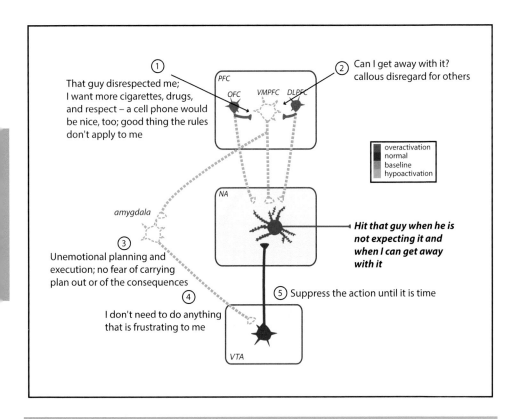

FIGURE 2.9. In psychopathic aggression, often seen in individuals with ASPD and conduct disorder, 1 and 2) the PFC is hypoactive, as it is in impulsive and psychotic aggression. Unlike in other forms of aggression, 3) the limbic system, including the amygdala, is hypoactive in psychopathic aggression. 4) Activation of the VTA is more controlled in psychopathic individuals, allowing them to 5) calculate the best time to act out with violence or aggression without consequences. The hypoactivation of the amygdala seen in psychopathically aggressive individuals is hypothesized to represent a paucity of fear conditioning (Rothemund et al., 2012). Thus, psychopathic individuals lack the ability to accurately predict impending harm from signals of threat and are unable to flexibly adjust to changes in reinforcement. This may explain why these patients never seem to develop a conscience.

Reduced Gray Matter Volume in Patients With ASPD and Psychopathy

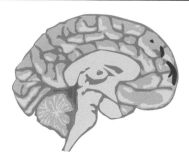 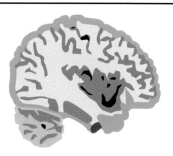

Anterior Rostral Medial Prefrontal Cortex
- Self-reflective processing
    - Facilitates other-person perspective
    - Enables emotional understanding of others' intentional acts

- Concurrent maintenance of 2 sets of competing information
    - Facilitates simultaneous consideration of self and other-person perspectives

- Engaged during fear appraisal

Temporal Poles
- Use stored conceptual knowledge and contextual framing
    - Facilitates understanding of social stimuli within a wider semantic and emotional context

FIGURE 2.10. Individuals with antisocial personality disorder and psychopathy (ASPD+P) have reduced gray matter volume in both the anterior rostral medial prefrontal cortex (arMPFC) and the temporal poles compared to individuals with antisocial personality disorder and no psychopathy (ASPD-P) (areas indicated in red) (Gregory et al., 2012). The arMPFC and the temporal poles function together to facilitate our understanding of others' emotional experiences and our awareness of how we are perceived by others. Structural abnormalities in these 2 brain areas may therefore contribute to the social impairments seen in patients with psychopathy and provide potential therapeutic targets for ameliorating violent behavior in these patients.

Mechanisms of Aggression in Different Psychiatric Disorders

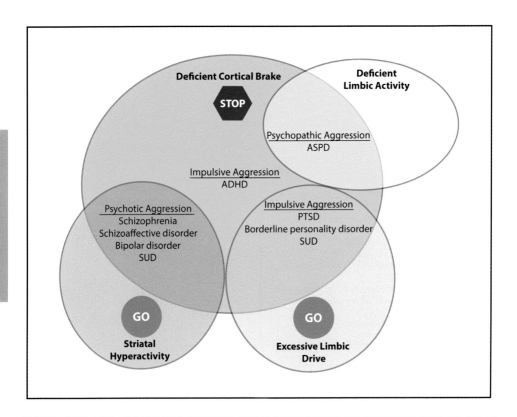

FIGURE 2.11. Supporting the proposed heterogeneous nature of violence and aggression, impaired neurocircuitry hypothetically varies among psychiatric disorders. Psychotic aggression, as seen in schizophrenia, theoretically results from hypoactivity in the PFC coupled with hyperactivity in the striatum, whereas impulsive aggression, as seen in borderline personality disorder, theoretically results from a combination of impaired top-down cortical control and hyperactive limbic drive. Psychopathic aggression, as exhibited in individuals with ASPD, hypothetically stems from hypoactive cortical control and hypoactive limbic drive. Given the varied impairments in neurocircuitry evident in impulsive, psychotic, and psychopathic aggression, it is not surprising that treatment strategies must also vary depending on the type of aggression being treated.

Neurotransmitter Systems Involved in Aggression

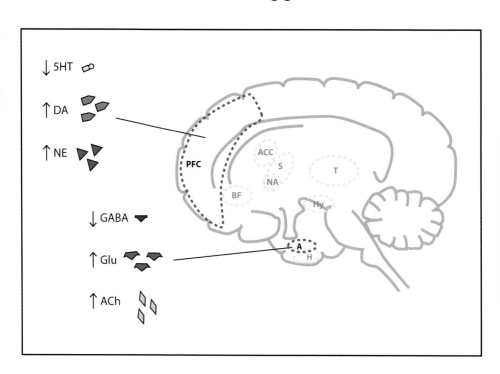

FIGURE 2.12. The neurotransmitters dopamine (DA), norepinephrine (NE), serotonin (5HT), acetylcholine (ACh), glutamate (Glu), and gamma-aminobutyric acid (GABA) are all thought to be involved in aggressive behavior. In the prefrontal cortex (PFC) of aggressive patients, 5HT is decreased, whereas both DA and NE are increased. In the amygdala (A) of aggressive patients, Glu and ACh are hypothetically increased, whereas GABA is decreased. Nonetheless, it is not surprising that the same neurotransmitter systems implicated in aggressive behavior, especially DA, 5HT, and GABA/Glu, are also thought to be altered in schizophrenia and other mental illnesses (Siever, 2008).

Dopamine and Aggression

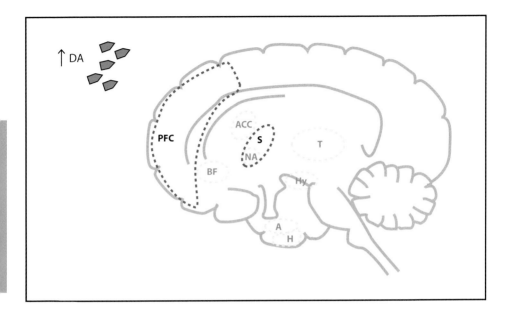

FIGURE 2.13. Dopamine (DA) is involved in the initiation and performance of aggressive behavior. Elevated levels of striatal and prefrontal cortical DA have been reported in individuals with impulsive disorders; this hyperdopaminergia may weaken the inhibitory pathways that regulate impulsivity (Siever, 2008).

Serotonin and Aggression

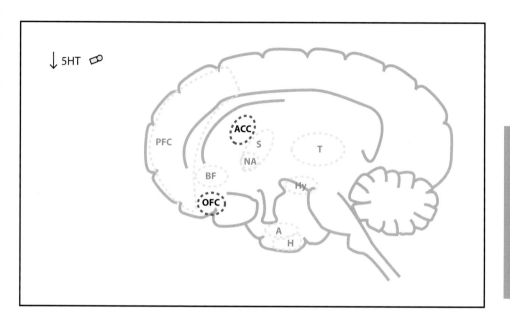

FIGURE 2.14. Serotonin (5HT) modulates prefrontal activity; thus, the serotonergic dysfunction observed in the OFC and the ACC of aggressive patients suggests a lack of sufficient top-down control (Siever, 2008). In fact, during aggressive confrontations, 5HT levels in the PFC may decrease by as much as 80% (Comai et al., 2012a). Aggressive behavior and suicide by violent means has been correlated with low cerebrospinal fluid (CSF) levels of 5H1AA, a measure of 5HT concentration. Additionally, whereas 5HT depletion increases aggressive behavior, increasing 5HT levels brings about increased activity in the PFC as well as diminished aggression (Coccaro et al., 2011).

Serotonin Receptors and Aggression

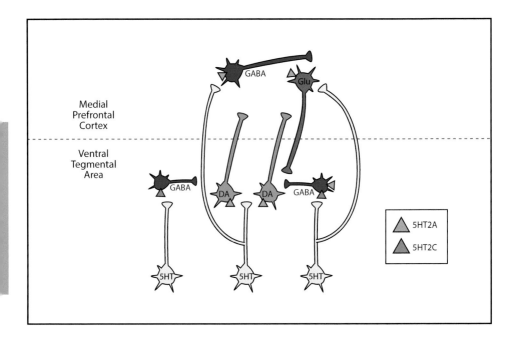

FIGURE 2.15. The serotonin 5HT2A receptor in particular may be implicated in aggressive behavior. The availability of the 5HT2A receptor in the OFC is hypothetically greater in aggressive patients with a comorbid personality disorder than in nonaggressive patients and healthy controls (Rosell et al., 2010). Contrary to the antiaggressive consequences of antagonism at 5HT2A receptors, agonism at 5HT2C receptors has been shown to reduce impulsivity (Winstanley et al., 2004). Both increased activity at 5HT2A receptors and decreased activity at 5HT2C receptors have been linked to aggressive behavior. Therefore, the targeting of specific serotonergic subtypes, a feature of many atypical antipsychotics, has potential for antiaggressive therapies.

GABA, Glutamate, and Aggression

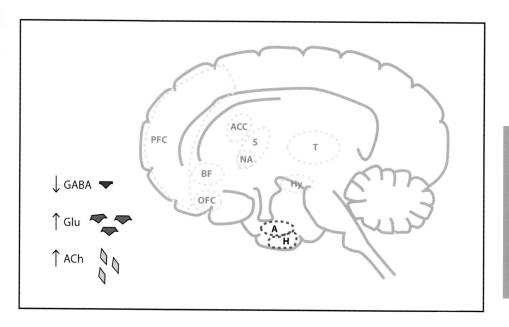

FIGURE 2.16. In limbic areas, including the hippocampus (H) and amygdala (A), GABA is hypothetically reduced, whereas Glu and ACh are hypothetically elevated. An imbalance of GABAergic and glutamatergic neurotransmission appears to contribute to the hyperactivity of limbic regions (Siever, 2008).

Acetylcholine and Aggression

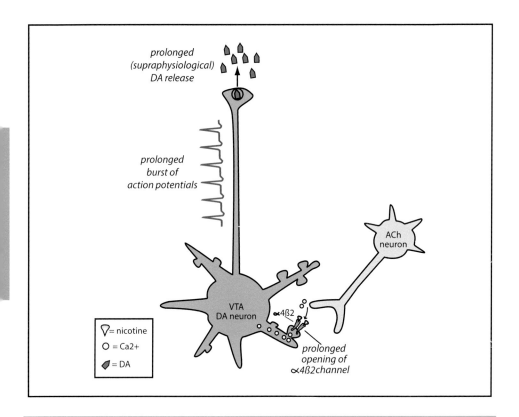

FIGURE 2.17. The binding of ACh to nicotinic receptors (nAChR) may increase impulsivity due at least in part to the promotion of DA release in the PFC and the ventral striatum (Ohmura et al., 2012). Nicotine is a full agonist at alpha-4 beta-2 nicotinic receptors located on DA neurons in the VTA and causes prolonged opening of nicotinic channels until they desensitize. This prolonged channel opening results in a prolonged burst of action potentials and consequently prolonged (supraphysiological) DA release. However, the role of ACh in aggressive behavior is not yet clear, as demonstrated by a recent study showing that the administration of a nicotine replacement patch reduced impulsive behavior in patients with schizophrenia (Barr et al., 2008). These contrasting data may be partially due to the pro-cognitive effects of ACh given that cognitive dysfunction has been linked to violent and aggressive behavior in patients with schizophrenia (Barr et al., 2008; Krakowski et al., 1989). Ca^2+: calcium

Can Aggressive Behavior Be Inherited?

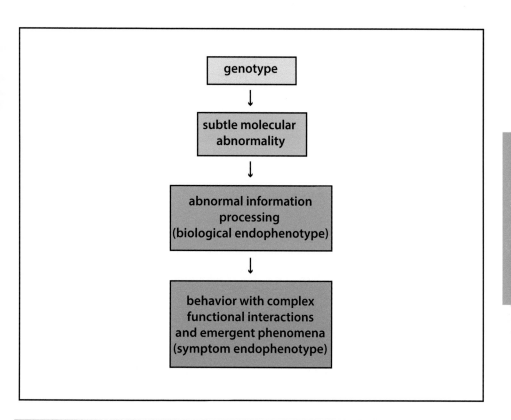

FIGURE 2.18. Data from twin and family studies indicate that violent behavior, especially impulsive aggression, is highly heritable (Siever, 2008). As with virtually all mental health issues, there is no one particular mutation associated with violent or aggressive behavior. Aggression is a complex, multifactorial trait that depends on the interaction between genetic components and environmental factors. Interestingly, many of the genetic polymorphisms associated with aggression depend on childhood experiences such as emotional trauma, indicating a neurodevelopmental process by which genes (i.e., nature) set up a risk component for aggressive behavior that becomes a reality only if certain adverse environmental factors (i.e., nurture) are encountered (Zammit et al., 2004).

MAO-A: The Warrior Gene

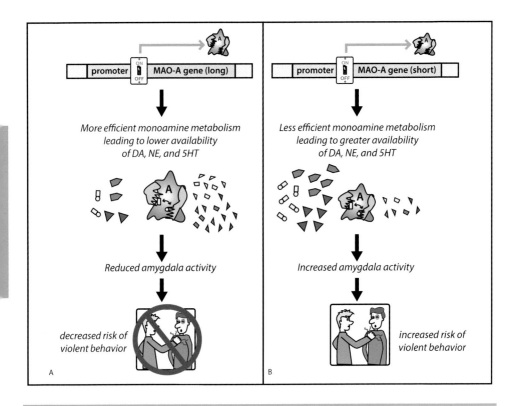

FIGURE 2.19. The gene for monoamine oxidase A (MAO-A) has been referred to as "the warrior gene" and has a very interesting relationship to aggressive behavior (Fergusson et al., 2011; McDermott et al., 2009). There are both short, low activity and long, high activity alleles of the MAO-A gene. The low activity variant has been associated with aggression in patients with schizophrenia. Since the MAO enzyme is involved in the degradation of monoamines, A) the long MAO-A allele gives rise to lower monoamine levels, whereas B) the short allele is associated with elevated monoamine levels that may lead to enhanced amygdala activity and increased aggression.

Testosterone Regulation of MAO-A Expression

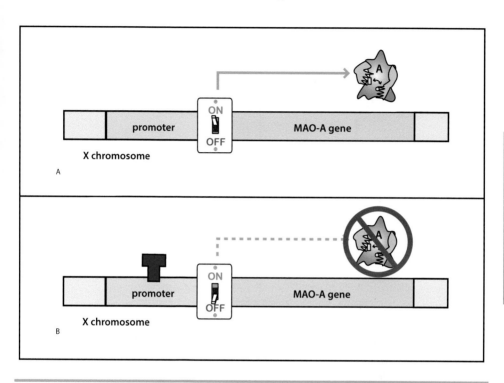

FIGURE 2.20. A) There is an androgen response element in the promoter region of the MAO-A gene; B) testosterone regulates the levels of MAO-A protein by binding to this response element (Sjoberg et al., 2008; Wu et al., 2009). Thus, testosterone levels could theoretically regulate MAO-A activity—and via this mechanism, aggression (see pages 14-17).

MAO-A, Child Abuse, and Sexual Dimorphism

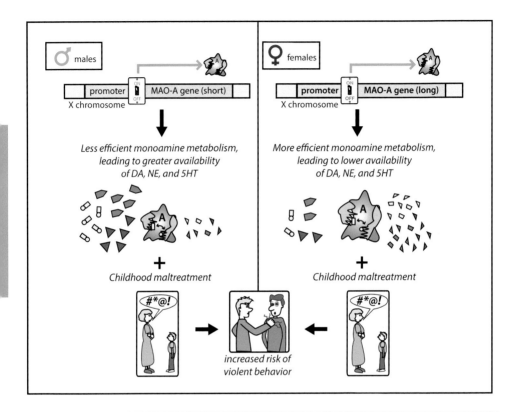

FIGURE 2.21. In males exposed to maltreatment as children, aggression is linked to the short, low activity allele; however, in females exposed to childhood maltreatment, it is the long, high activity allele that correlates with aggressive behavior (Aslund et al., 2011). This gene X environment X sex relationship with aggression is especially fascinating given that the MAO-A gene is located on the X chromosome and therefore present in twice the number of chromosomes in women than in men.

MAO-A Polymorphisms and Impulsivity

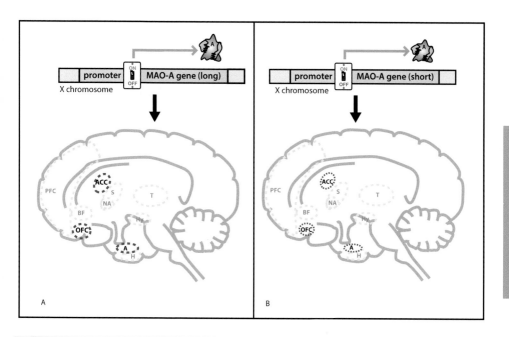

FIGURE 2.22. Compared to A) healthy men with the long, high activity variant of the MAO-A gene, B) healthy men with the short, low activity variant of the MAO-A gene have structural and functional differences in key brain areas associated with impulsive behavior, including the OFC, the amygdala, and the ACC. Although this study by Meyer-Lindenberg et al. (2006) was performed in healthy individuals, the data suggest that variation in the MAO-A gene may present a genetic bias toward impulsivity and aggression.

COMT and Aggression

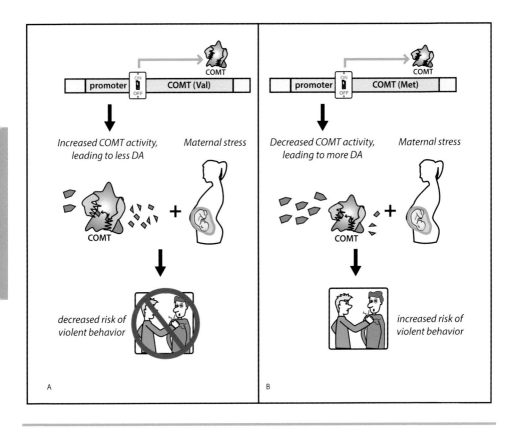

FIGURE 2.23. A) Along with NE, catechol-O-methyltransferase (COMT) is one of the key enzymes involved in the degradation of DA, especially in the PFC. B) Individuals with the Met/Met COMT genotype have 5-fold lower COMT activity than those with the Val/Val genotype. Men with 2 copies of the Met allele may be at an increased risk of impulsive behavior and conduct problems compared to Val homozygotes, but only following exposure to maternal stress in utero (Thompson et al., 2012).

5HTTLPR and Aggression

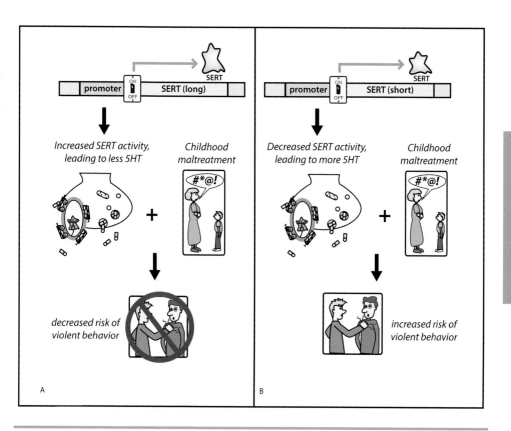

FIGURE 2.24. A) Genetic variation in the serotonin transporter gene 5HTTLPR has been linked with increased amygdala activation, impulsive behavior, and violent suicide in schizophrenia (Bayle et al., 2003). B) The short variant of 5HTTLPR leads to the expression of a less efficient serotonin reuptake transporter (SERT) that is associated with reduced 5HT uptake and thus greater synaptic 5HT concentration. This short variant of 5HTTLPR is associated with an increased risk of impulsive aggressive behavior (Retz et al., 2004). It has been proposed that the increase in 5HT may disturb neurocircuitry during development, resulting in impaired serotonergic neurotransmission (Meyer-Lindenberg et al., 2006). As with many of the other genetic polymorphisms correlated with violence and aggression, the association appears to depend on childhood maltreatment (Cicchetti et al., 2012).

Summary of Genes Associated With Violence and Aggression

Gene	Variant Associated With Violence and Aggression	Proposed Neurobiological Consequence
MAO-A	Short allele in males	Increased monoamines
	Long allele in females	Decreased monoamines
COMT	Met allele	Increased dopamine
5HTTLPR	Short allele	Increased 5HT levels during neurodevelopment
FKBP5	H2 haplotype	Impaired glucocorticoid receptor response to cortisol leading to heightened HPA axis response to stress

FIGURE 2.25. Given the increased risk of violence and aggression in the schizophrenia population, it may be that the same genetic polymorphisms that increase one's risk of developing a mental illness such as schizophrenia or bipolar disorder also increase one's risk of impulsive tendencies. The neurobiological dysfunction underlying symptoms of mental illness may also impair one's ability to control impulsive responses or empathize with others. However, taken together, the studies of genetic factors associated with violent and aggressive behavior elucidate the neurobiological substrates underlying violence and aggression. Additionally, these studies suggest that in conjunction with a detailed patient history that includes childhood experiences, screening for genetic risk factors may help clinicians identify patients with schizophrenia and other mental illnesses who are at an increased risk of violence and aggression.

| Chapter 3

Treatment of Violence and Aggression

Given the enormous consequences of violent and aggressive behavior, we are in great need of effective treatment strategies that can reduce violence and aggression. Unfortunately, most research trials exclude patients who are violent or aggressive, so establishing the best treatment strategy for these patients is difficult and must rely in part upon clinical experience. Chapter 3 aims to explain the options available for the treatment of violence and aggression, including antipsychotics (including high-dose antipsychotic treatment), mood stabilizers, antidepressants, stimulants, adrenergic blockers, opiate antagonists, and benzodiazepines. It is important to note that there is no FDA-approved agent for the treatment of chronic aggression; thus, all of the treatment strategies described in this chapter should be initiated with not only caution, but also documented patient consent whenever possible.

Antiaggression Treatments: Dampening Bottom-Up Drive and Enhancing Top-Down Brakes

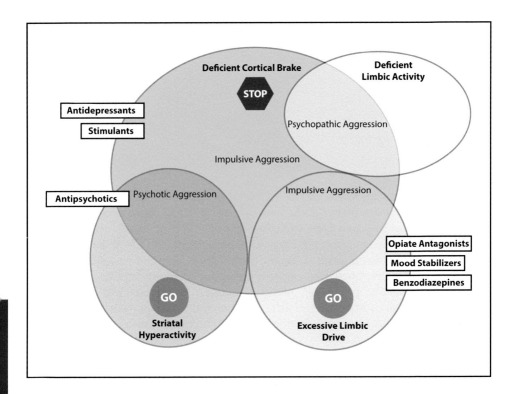

FIGURE 3.1. Aggression is heterogeneous in nature, and each type of aggression (impulsive, psychotic, and psychopathic) may be attributable to dysfunction in a different neural circuit. It is therefore not surprising that effective treatment strategies for aggressive behavior must be tailored to target the underlying neural dysfunction. For example, antidepressants (namely, serotonin reuptake inhibitors) and stimulants may improve the deficiencies in top-down cortical control evident in impulsive aggression, whereas antipsychotics may be able to address both the impaired top-down cortical control and excessive drive from striatal hyperactivity that are seen in psychotic aggression.

Antipsychotics for the Treatment of Violence and Aggression

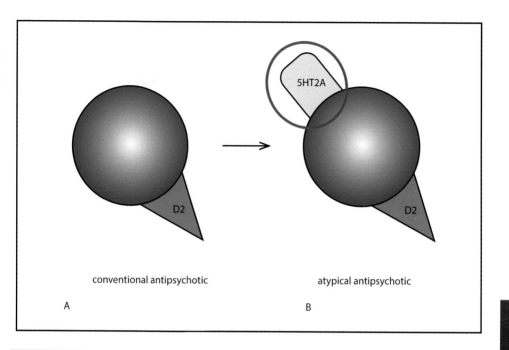

5HT2A

D2

D2

conventional antipsychotic

atypical antipsychotic

A

B

FIGURE 3.2. There is still some debate as to whether antipsychotics are effective for the treatment of violence in general or only for violent behavior associated with psychosis. However, substantial practice-based evidence from forensic settings suggests that antipsychotics, most notably clozapine and olanzapine, may be effective in treating many patients with psychotic or impulsive aggression (Frogley et al., 2012; Krakowski et al., 2006; Swanson et al., 2008). Of the antiaggressive treatment options available, including mood stabilizers and antidepressants, antipsychotics have the largest evidence base in terms of efficacy. A) First-generation, conventional antipsychotics bind primarily to and block dopamine D2 receptors, leading to a reduction in dopaminergic neurotransmission throughout the brain. B) Second-generation, atypical antipsychotics also act as antagonists at D2 receptors but have the additional property of blocking serotonin 5HT2A receptors. This 5HT2A antagonism is thought to temper some of the adverse effects (e.g., extrapyramidal symptoms) caused by D2 antagonism.

Dopamine D2 Receptor Occupancy

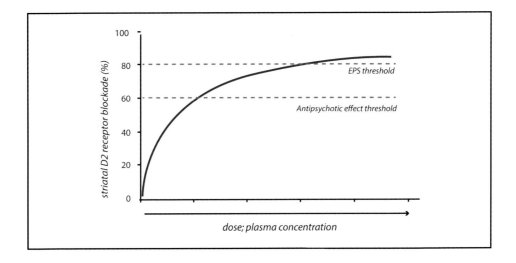

FIGURE 3.3. Antipsychotic blockade of at least 60% of D2 receptors in the striatum is necessary to ameliorate psychotic symptoms. However, when 80% or more of D2 receptors are blocked, extrapyramidal symptoms (EPS) are likely to occur. Standard doses of atypical antipsychotics are based on achieving 60% D2 receptor occupancy without exceeding the 80% EPS threshold. Note that the slope of the curve flattens out with increasing dose; that is, at higher doses, large increases in dose are needed to obtain substantial increases in D2 receptor occupancy.

Pharmacokinetics and Pharmacodynamics

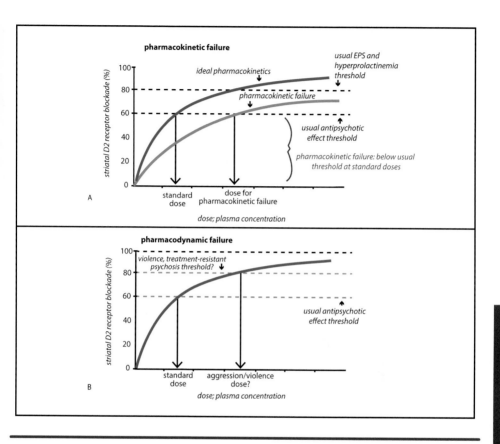

FIGURE 3.4. The failure of a patient to respond to antipsychotic treatment may be due to either pharmacokinetic or pharmacodynamic failure. A) Pharmacokinetic failure occurs in cases in which the therapeutic threshold (~60% D2 occupancy) is not achieved despite dosing at standard therapeutic levels. B) Pharmacodynamic failure occurs in cases in which occupancy of greater than 80% of D2 receptors may be required before therapeutic effects are achieved. Pharmacodynamic failure therefore alters antipsychotics' threshold for therapeutic effects and may be quite prevalent in patients with psychotic or impulsive aggression.

High-Dose Monotherapy and Antipsychotic Polypharmacy

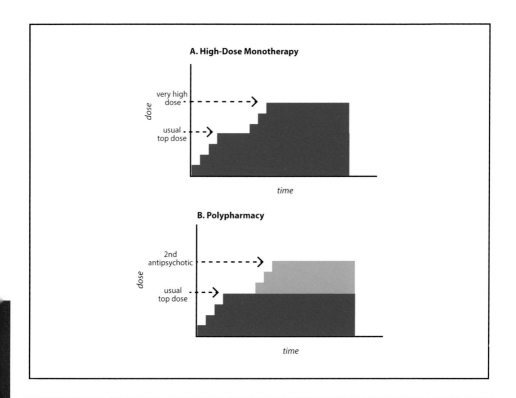

FIGURE 3.5. For patients who are psychotically aggressive and continue to exhibit violent behavior despite adequate trials of antipsychotic monotherapies, it may be necessary to employ strategies aimed at overcoming pharmacokinetic or pharmacodynamic failure. In such cases, there are essentially 2 treatment strategies that can increase D2 receptor occupancy: high-dose antipsychotic monotherapy and antipsychotic polypharmacy. A) High-dose monotherapy involves increasing the dose beyond standard therapeutic levels using slow uptitration. B) In polypharmacy, a second antipsychotic is added to antipsychotic monotherapy; both agents are dosed at standard therapeutic levels. Several studies have reported that neither high-dose monotherapy nor polypharmacy is more efficacious for the "average" patient; however, there is some consensus that a subpopulation, including individuals who are violent, may require such heroic measures.

Defining an Adequate Antipsychotic Trial: Time as a Drug

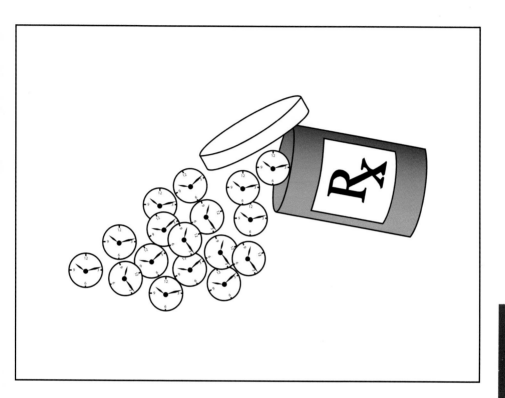

FIGURE 3.6. The downstream effects of D2 receptor blockade may take more than 6 weeks to manifest in some patients. In such cases, time may act as a drug (Morrissette and Stahl, 2012). Oftentimes, a second antipsychotic is added to the first when there is an inadequate response after only a few weeks of monotherapy. Adding a second antipsychotic may therefore be superfluous, increasing the monetary and side effect burdens of treatment without any additional therapeutic benefit.

Treatment Algorithm for the Use of Antipsychotics

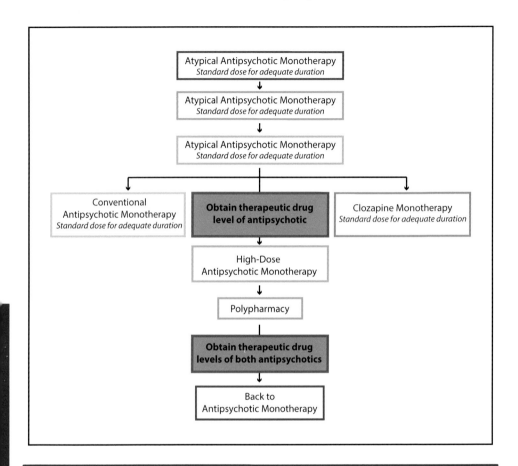

FIGURE 3.7. Despite several guidelines recommending that antipsychotic polypharmacy be employed only as a last resort (following the failure of several antipsychotic monotherapies and a trial of clozapine), many clinicians attempt polypharmacy as the rule rather than the exception. Polypharmacy may be useful for overcoming pharmacokinetic and pharmacodynamic failure and recruiting additional receptor binding properties that may be useful for treating nonpsychotic symptoms such as anxiety and depression. However, each antipsychotic also binds receptors associated with adverse effects, so the side effect burden may be increased when polypharmacy is used. Importantly, therapeutic drug levels should be monitored, especially before attempting high-dose monotherapy or antipsychotic polypharmacy.

Vast Molecular Polypharmacy
of Atypical Antipsychotics

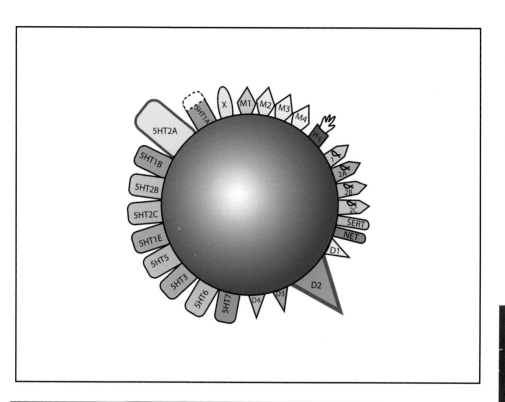

FIGURE 3.8. The atypical antipsychotics were developed as a means to block D2 receptors while avoiding some of the negative consequences of excessive and indiscriminate D2 receptor antagonism. All atypical antipsychotics bind 5HT2A as well as D2 receptors. The antagonism of 5HT2A receptors tempers some of the effects of D2 receptor antagonism, potentially reducing the development of EPS. Atypical antipsychotics bind to other receptors in addition to D2 and 5HT2A; each agent has a unique binding profile that lends it additional therapeutic and adverse effects. Although atypical antipsychotics as a class have less propensity to cause EPS than conventional antipsychotics, there is an increased risk of cardiometabolic issues with many atypical antipsychotics.

Molecular Binding Profiles of Atypical Antipsychotics

Drug	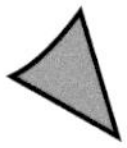 D2 Antag	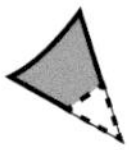 D2 PA	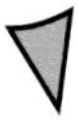 D3	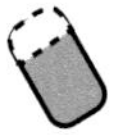 5HT1A	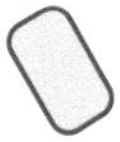 5HT2A
Aripiprazole		+++	+++	+++	++
Asenapine	+++		+++	++	++++
Clozapine	+		+	+	+
Iloperidone	+++		++	++	+++
Lurasidone	+++		?	+++	++
Olanzapine	++		++		+++
Paliperidone	+++		+++	+	++++
Quetiapine	+		+	+*	++*
Risperidone	+++		+++	+	++++
Ziprasidone	+++		+++	++	++++
Therapeutic Effects	Reduced positive symptoms	Reduced positive symptoms	Reduced positive symptoms; Reduced negative symptoms; Procognitive; Antidepressant	Reduced EPS; Reduced hyperprolactinemia; Antidepressant; Anxiolytic	Reduced EPS; Reduced hyperprolactinemia
Side Effects	EPS; Hyperprolactinemia; Increased negative symptoms; Increased cognitive deficits; Sedation	Relatively lower risk of EPS	Unknown	Unknown	Cardiometabolic

+ weak binding affinity (100>Ki<1000)
++ moderate binding affinity (10>Ki<100)
+++ strong binding affinity (1>Ki<10)
++++ very strong binding affinity (Ki<1)
? no data yet available
* binding property due primarily to the metabolite norquetiapine

FIGURE 3.9. The binding affinities for various receptors hypothetically give each atypical antipsychotic a unique therapeutic and side effect profile (NIMH Psychoactive Drug Screening Program).

5HT2C	5HT7	α1	M1	M3	H1
++	+++	++			++
++++	++++	+++	+		+++
+	++	+++	+++	++	+++
+	++	+++			++
+	++++	++			
++	+	++	++	++	+++
++	+++	+++			++
+*	++*	+++	++*	++*	+++*
++	+++	+++			++
++	+++	++			++
Antidepressant	Reduced circadian rhythm dysfunction; Reduced negative symptoms; Procognitive	Reduced nightmares	Reduced EPS	Reduced EPS	Hypnotic
Cardiometabolic	Unknown	Dizziness; Sedation; Hypotension	Constipation; Sedation; Dry mouth; Blurred vision	Cardiometabolic; Constipation; Sedation; Dry mouth; Blurred vision	Cardiometabolic; Sedation

Receptor Binding Affinities Relative to Dopamine D2

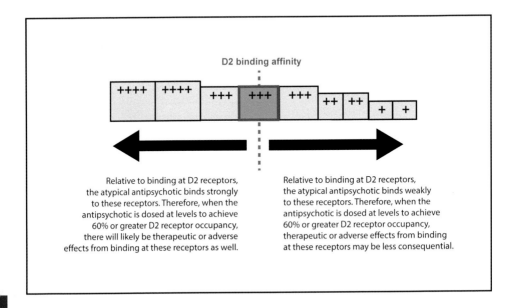

D2 binding affinity

| ++++ | ++++ | +++ | +++ | +++ | ++ | ++ | + | + |

Relative to binding at D2 receptors, the atypical antipsychotic binds strongly to these receptors. Therefore, when the antipsychotic is dosed at levels to achieve 60% or greater D2 receptor occupancy, there will likely be therapeutic or adverse effects from binding at these receptors as well.

Relative to binding at D2 receptors, the atypical antipsychotic binds weakly to these receptors. Therefore, when the antipsychotic is dosed at levels to achieve 60% or greater D2 receptor occupancy, therapeutic or adverse effects from binding at these receptors may be less consequential.

FIGURE 3.10. With the exception of clozapine, antipsychotics are dosed at a level that blocks 60-80% of D2 receptors. It is important to note that any receptor binding that is stronger than that of D2 receptors will also be occupied at levels greater than 60% and will likely cause additional therapeutic and adverse effects. It is essential to keep the relative receptor binding affinities in mind when dosing an atypical antipsychotic at higher than usual levels to attain greater than 80% occupancy of D2 receptors so that the potential effects of binding to receptors other than D2 receptors can be anticipated and monitored. On the following pages, graphical representations of each atypical antipsychotic's binding affinities relative to D2 are shown. To the left of D2 are the receptors that an antipsychotic binds to with more affinity than for D2; to the right are the receptors that an antipsychotic binds to with weaker affinity than for D2.

High-Dose Monotherapy: Clozapine

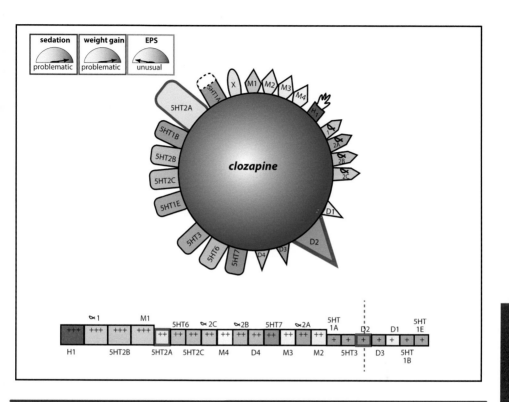

FIGURE 3.11. Although clozapine is not recommended as a first-line treatment due to the risk of serious adverse effects (most notably agranulocytosis) in patients who have failed several first-line atypical antipsychotic monotherapies, a trial of clozapine is recommended. The efficacy of clozapine has been well documented in treatment-resistant patients and those who are violent or aggressive. Interestingly, the antiaggressive effects of clozapine are somewhat independent of its ability to improve positive symptoms of psychosis; thus, clozapine may be a useful treatment for nonpsychotic aggression and is recommended first line for the treatment of persistently aggressive behavior. Usual doses of clozapine (plasma levels of 400-600 ng/mL) actually bind less than 60-80% of D2 receptors. However, clozapine often has antipsychotic effects at 20-67% D2 occupancy, suggesting that the antipsychotic effects of clozapine go beyond its ability to block D2 receptors. This is not surprising given the vast binding profile of clozapine.

High-Dose Monotherapy: Olanzapine

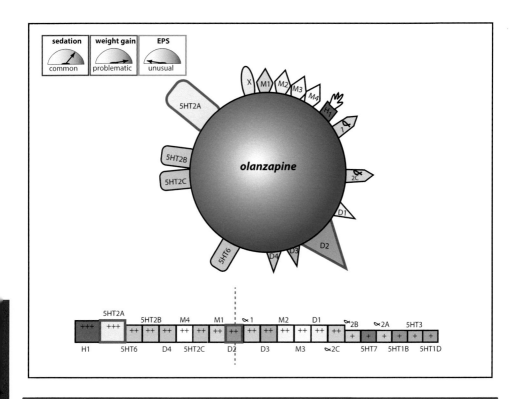

FIGURE 3.12. A substantial body of evidence supports the use of olanzapine for the treatment of aggression. It has been postulated that the antiaggressive effects of olanzapine may be due at least in part to its procognitive effects. Olanzapine is a good alternative in cases in which clozapine cannot be used. Olanzapine is perhaps the most well-studied atypical antipsychotic in terms of its use at high doses. The risk of EPS is minimal with olanzapine, even at high doses; however, among the atypical antipsychotics, olanzapine carries one of the greatest risks of cardiometabolic effects, perhaps due in part to its strong binding affinity for histaminic H1 and serotonin 5HT2C receptors. Olanzapine may be most effective at higher doses (40-60 mg/day) and may be useful in treatment-resistant violent patients in forensic settings at doses as high as 60-90 mg/day. Olanzapine titration to higher doses should take place with dose escalation every 5-7 days. Olanzapine is also available in a long-acting depot formulation that can be supplemented with oral olanzapine to achieve high D2 receptor occupancy.

High-Dose Monotherapy: Risperidone

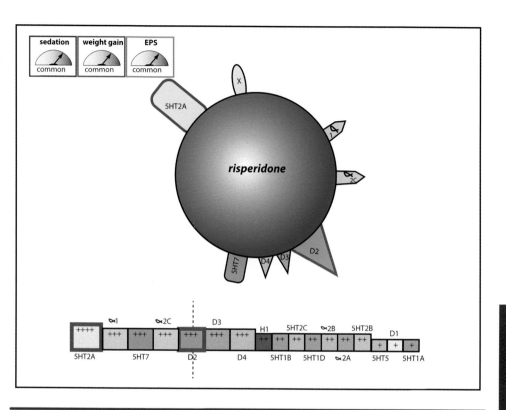

FIGURE 3.13. Risperidone has also shown significant efficacy in reducing aggression and hostility in various patient populations, including schizophrenia, developmental disorders, autism, and disruptive behavior disorder. In the "average" patient, the dosing of risperidone at 2-4 mg/day is associated with 70-80% D2 receptor occupancy, and risperidone is rarely useful at doses above 8 mg/day. Both risperidone and paliperidone are associated with an increased risk of EPS in a dose-dependent manner, so care must be exercised when increasing the doses of these agents. The titration of risperidone to high doses should be executed by increasing the dose every 5-7 days. Risperidone is also available in a long-acting depot formulation, so an alternative strategy for achieving high D2 receptor occupancy is the simultaneous use of the depot formulation and oral risperidone.

High-Dose Monotherapy: Paliperidone

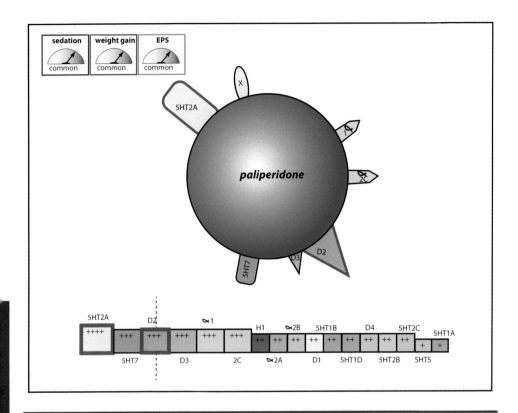

FIGURE 3.14. Paliperidone is the active metabolite of risperidone and has a similar receptor binding profile with relatively strong affinity for D2 receptors. One pharmacokinetic difference between risperidone and paliperidone is that the latter is not metabolized in the liver, so it has a smaller chance of drug-drug interactions or effects from cytochrome P450 polymorphisms. Paliperidone may also be more tolerable, with less sedation and fewer EPS, and it should be dosed higher than risperidone. The titration of paliperidone to high doses should be executed by increasing the dose every 5-7 days. Paliperidone is also available in a long-acting depot formulation that may be used in combination with oral paliperidone to achieve high D2 receptor occupancy.

High-Dose Monotherapy: Quetiapine

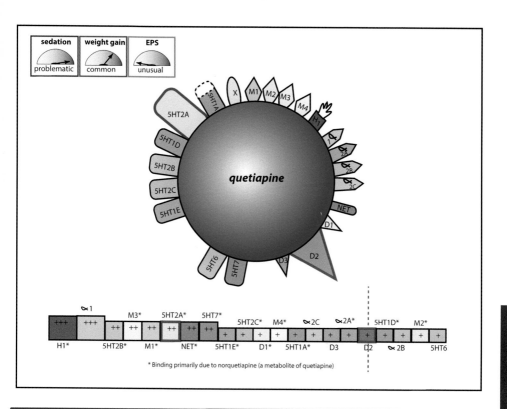

FIGURE 3.15. Quetiapine has been shown to be effective for the treatment of aggression associated with schizophrenia, bipolar disorder, attention deficit hyperactivity disorder (ADHD), and borderline personality disorder. Quetiapine binds D2 receptors with relatively weak affinity; it has far greater affinity for many other receptors. Because of this binding profile, high doses of at least 800 mg/day are usually required for quetiapine to have antipsychotic effects. Quetiapine carries a very low risk of EPS, even at high doses, but it is associated with a moderate risk of sedation and metabolic syndrome, perhaps due in part to its high binding affinity for H1 and 5HT2C receptors. The use of quetiapine in forensic settings at doses up to 1800 mg/day may be effective in violent patients who tolerate but do not respond to lower doses. The titration of quetiapine usually involves daily dose increases, but the dose should be increased at a slower rate when exceeding 800 mg/day.

High-Dose Monotherapy: Ziprasidone

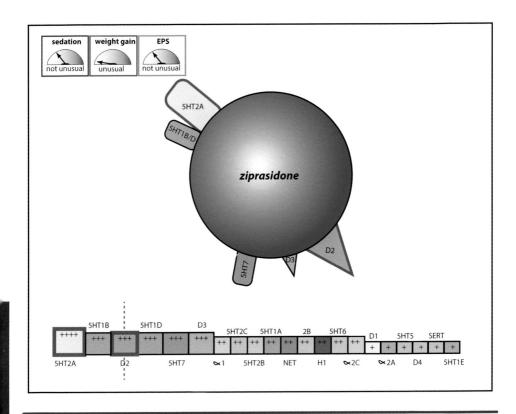

FIGURE 3.16. Ziprasidone may be effective for treating aggression and has been shown to work quite rapidly when administered in its intramuscular formulation. Ziprasidone has a fairly high binding affinity for D2 receptors; this affinity is surpassed only by its affinity for serotonin 5HT2A and 5HT1B receptors. Ziprasidone is associated with virtually no risk of metabolic effects, and earlier concerns about QTc prolongation have not been supported. Importantly, ziprasidone must be taken with food in order to optimize its absorption. Higher doses of ziprasidone may be most effective, and doses as high as 360 mg/day have been reported. Ziprasidone can be titrated to high doses with daily dose increases.

High-Dose Monotherapy: Aripiprazole

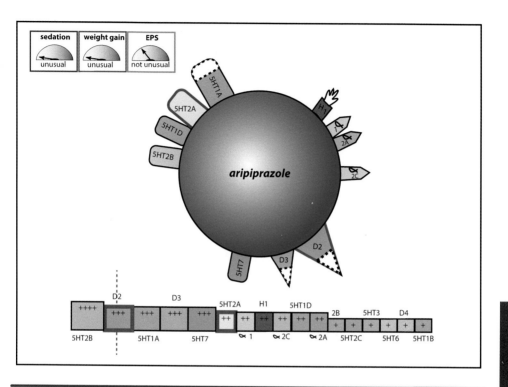

FIGURE 3.17. Some data indicate that aripiprazole has antiaggressive effects in patients with schizophrenia. Aripiprazole is a unique member of the atypical antipsychotic drug class. Rather than acting as a D2 receptor antagonist, aripiprazole acts as a partial agonist at D2 receptors. This means that in the presence of a full D2 receptor agonist (e.g., dopamine), aripiprazole acts as an antagonist at D2 receptors; however, in the absence of a D2 receptor agonist, aripiprazole acts as a net agonist at D2 receptors. Due to its very high binding affinity for D2 receptors compared to other antipsychotics, in the presence of a D2 receptor antagonist (e.g., another antipsychotic), aripiprazole can potentially reverse the actions of the other antipsychotic. Given its partial agonism and its very high binding affinity for D2 receptors, aripiprazole may actually be less effective in treating psychosis at higher doses and may reduce the effectiveness of another antipsychotic if an attempt at polypharmacy is made. Aripiprazole is not associated with a significant risk of sedation, EPS, or metabolic syndrome but may cause akathisia. Although the initial titration of aripiprazole can be rapid, dose increases after a steady state has been reached should be done every 10-14 days.

High-Dose Monotherapy: Iloperidone

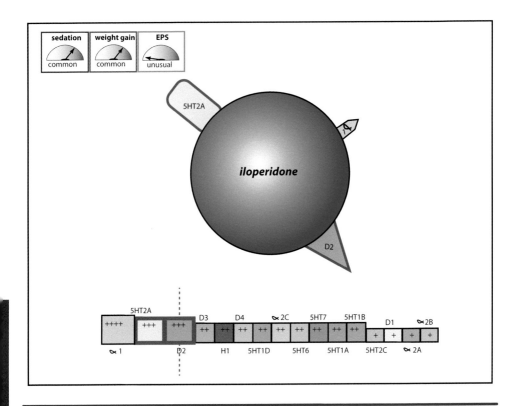

FIGURE 3.18. Iloperidone, asenapine, and lurasidone are the newest atypical antipsychotics on the market, so less is known about their uses at high doses. When attempting to use a high-dose strategy, it would be prudent to first try a high-dose trial of one of the older atypical antipsychotics that has more clinical experience. Iloperidone is distinguished by its high binding affinity for adrenergic alpha-1 receptors. Due to this binding property, iloperidone is associated with a high risk of orthostatic hypotension and sedation, so it must be titrated slowly and is not recommended for use at high doses.

High-Dose Monotherapy:
Asenapine

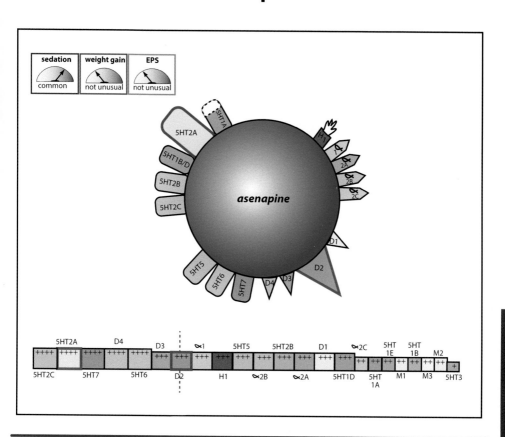

FIGURE 3.19. Asenapine has moderate binding affinity for D2 receptors and is usually not associated with an increased risk of EPS or metabolic syndrome. Asenapine is available only in a sublingual formulation and therefore may be a good option for patients who have pharmacokinetic failure in response to other antipsychotics due to hepatic metabolism or poor absorption. Doses as high as 30-40 mg/day can be used but must be administered 10 mg at a time, with doses given at least 1 hour apart. The titration of asenapine should be done by increasing the dose every 5-7 days.

High-Dose Monotherapy: Lurasidone

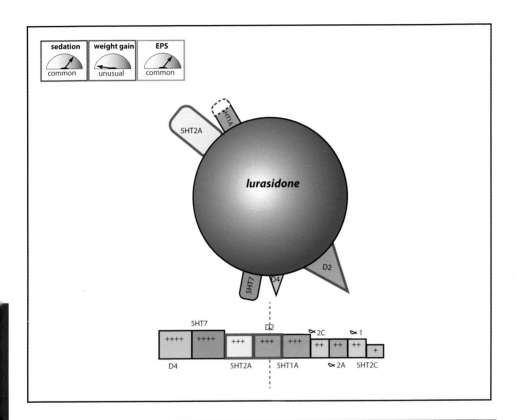

FIGURE 3.20. Lurasidone is the newest antipsychotic approved for use in the United States. It has moderately high binding affinity for D2 receptors but is notable for its antagonism of serotonin 5HT7 receptors. Lurasidone is approved up to 80 mg/ day but may be more effective in some patients at doses as high as 160 mg/day. Importantly, lurasidone should be taken with food to optimize absorption. Although the original trials of lurasidone suggested that the risk of side effects increased with higher dosing, recent data indicate that the administration of lurasidone in the evening may minimize the risk of side effects.

High-Dose Monotherapy: Guidelines for Atypical Antipsychotics

Medication	Usual Dose Range (mg/day)*	Considerations for High Dosing
Clozapine	300-450	Maximum dose is usually 900 mg/day; doses above 550 mg/day may require concomitant anticonvulsant administration to reduce the chances of a seizure
Risperidone	2-8	FDA-approved up to 16 mg/day; very high doses usually not tolerated
Paliperidone	3-6	Maximum dose is generally 12 mg/day
Olanzapine	10-20	Some forensic settings up to 90 mg/day
Quetiapine	300-750	Some forensic settings up to 1800 mg/day
Ziprasidone	80-160	Must be taken with food; PET data support >120 mg/day; some forensic settings up to 360 mg/day may be appropriate
Aripiprazole	10-30	Higher doses usually not more effective and possibly less effective
Iloperidone	12-24	High dosing not well studied and may be limited due to risk of orthostatic hypotension
Asenapine	10-20	High dosing not well studied
Lurasidone	40-160	Must be taken with food; nightly administration may improve tolerability; high dosing not well studied, but some patients may benefit from doses up to 160 mg/day

* Based on oral formulation in adults

FIGURE 3.21. As with all off-label practices, the dosing of antipsychotics above standard therapeutic levels warrants informed consent and increased monitoring of the patient. As pharmacokinetic and pharmacodynamic characteristics vary from patient to patient, it is virtually impossible to predict which daily dose will be needed to achieve an antipsychotic effect. Antipsychotic dosing should be started at the lowest FDA-approved level and then uptitrated until therapeutic efficacy or intolerable side effects occur.

High-Dose Monotherapy:
Conventional Antipsychotics

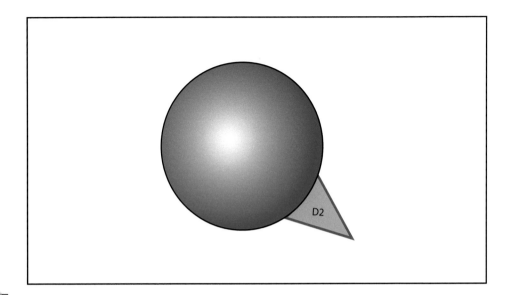

FIGURE 3.22. Conventional antipsychotics were designed to tightly bind D2 receptors and are effective in ameliorating psychotic symptoms for many patients. However, the indiscriminate antagonism of D2 receptors in the nigrostriatal and mesolimbic pathways often has disturbing motor effects, including EPS, akathisia, tardive dyskinesia, and hyperprolactinemia. Nevertheless, high-dose monotherapy using conventional antipsychotics is often surprisingly well tolerated. The strategy for achieving a high dose of these agents involves gradually increasing the dose beyond the upper limit of the dosing range and beyond the usual plasma drug levels. The risk of EPS, akathisia, tardive dyskinesia, and elevated prolactin must be part of the risk:benefit calculation when using any conventional antipsychotic. Haloperidol and fluphenazine may be preferable, as their blood levels are better understood and as they have injectable depot formulations available. Of note is the fact that some individuals may actually show increased aggression following treatment with a conventional antipsychotic such as haloperidol, especially at higher doses. This increase in aggression may be a manifestation of treatment-induced psychomotor agitation.

Mood Stabilizers

	Hypothetical Mechanism of Antiaggression			
	Increased serotonergic neurotransmission	Increased GABAergic neurotransmission	Decreased glutamatergic neurotransmission	Decreased dopaminergic neurotransmission
Anticonvulsants				
Valproate		✔	✔	
Lamotrigine			✔	
Topiramate		✔	✔	
Carbamazepine/ Oxcarbazepine		✔	✔	
Phenytoin	✔	✔	✔	
Lithium		✔	✔	✔

FIGURE 3.23. Mood stabilizers, including lithium and anticonvulsants, may alter the ratio of glutamate to GABA in limbic areas, reducing irritability and impulsivity. Many of these agents, including valproate, have historically been used as adjunctive medications for the treatment of impulsive aggression. More recent studies have found conflicting data regarding the benefit of adding a mood stabilizer to an antipsychotic in the treatment of aggression (Citrome et al., 2007). Nevertheless, this strategy may be effective for some patients who are impulsively aggressive. It is not fully understood whether the antiaggressive effects of anticonvulsants are secondary to mood stabilization or the calming of seizure-like hyperactivity of limbic regions and a reduction in bottom-up drive (Comai et al., 2012). With regard to the use of valproate in treating impulsive aggression, evidence suggests that it may be most effective during the first week of treatment, with diminishing effects thereafter (Citrome et al., 2004). When using topiramate to treat impulsive aggression, low doses should be employed, as the use of higher doses may actually exacerbate aggressive behavior. Similarly, for lithium, it may be best to maintain doses lower than those typically used in the treatment of bipolar mania (Comai et al., 2012).

Antidepressants

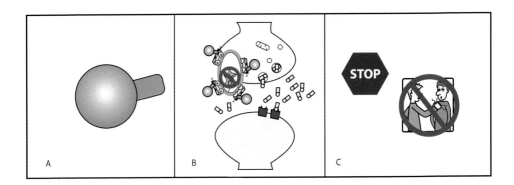

A   B   C

FIGURE 3.24. A) Selective serotonin reuptake inhibitors (SSRIs) as well as other antidepressants B) increase prefrontal cortical levels of 5HT by preventing its reuptake from the synapse. C) In theory, the increase in prefrontal 5HT may enhance top-down control of impulsive aggression, thereby facilitating the inhibition of subcortical areas. Several small studies have shown promise for the antiaggressive effects of the SSRIs fluoxetine, citalopram, and sertraline (Volavka and Citrome, 2012).

Stimulants

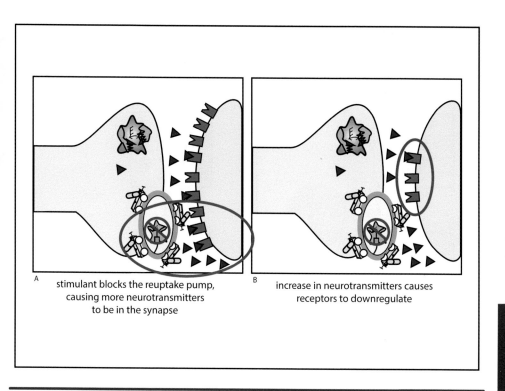

A — stimulant blocks the reuptake pump, causing more neurotransmitters to be in the synapse

B — increase in neurotransmitters causes receptors to downregulate

FIGURE 3.25. Stimulants increase dopamine (DA) and norepinephrine (NE) levels in the prefrontal cortex (PFC). Thus, it may seem paradoxical to treat aggression, in which DA and NE are hypothetically already elevated in the PFC, with stimulants. However, stimulants have been found to be effective in treating impulsive aggression, especially when associated with ADHD. A) Stimulants act by blocking the reuptake of NE and DA in the cortex, leading to increased levels of DA and NE in the synapse. B) With sustained treatment using a stimulant, postsynaptic NE and DA receptors are actually down-regulated or desensitized in response to the excess DA and NE. This down-regulation or desensitization is hypothesized to ultimately cause a reduction in excessive baseline dopaminergic and noradrenergic neurotransmission.

Adrenergic Blockers

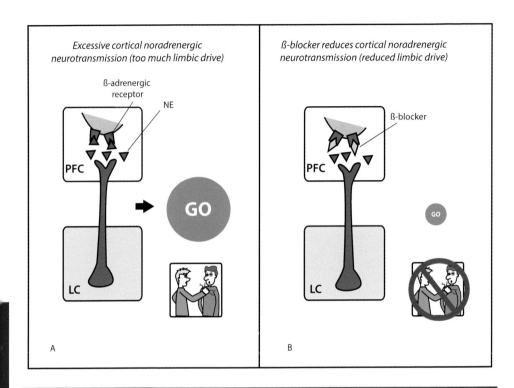

Excessive cortical noradrenergic neurotransmission (too much limbic drive)

ß-blocker reduces cortical noradrenergic neurotransmission (reduced limbic drive)

FIGURE 3.26. Beta-adrenergic blockers, including pindolol, propranolol, and nadolol, are often used as adjunctive treatments to control aggressive behavior in patients with schizophrenia. Beta-adrenergic blockers have propensity for cardiovascular side effects, so caution should be exercised when using these agents. A and B) Beta-adrenergic blockers may be particularly effective in patients who are violent or aggressive due to excessive NE levels and in individuals who are unresponsive to or intolerable of antipsychotics. Clonidine, which modifies noradrenergic transmission via antagonist actions at adrenergic alpha-2 receptors rather than beta-adrenergic receptors, has also been effectively used as an adjunctive treatment for aggression in patients with schizophrenia.

Opiate Antagonists

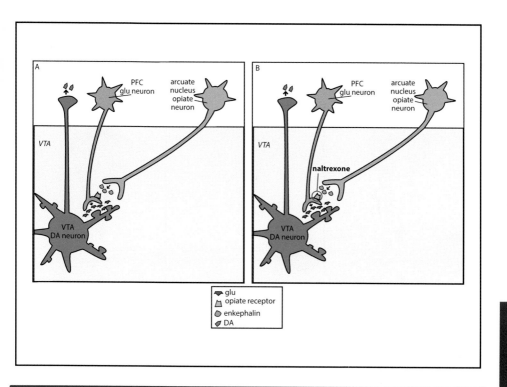

FIGURE 3.27. Opiate antagonists may also be useful for treating aggression. A) Endogenous opiates such as enkephalins activate presynaptic opiate receptors on glutamatergic projections in the ventral tegmental area (VTA). The excitation of dopaminergic neurons in the VTA leads to increased DA release in the PFC. B) Opiate antagonists such as naltrexone block the release of glutamate, leading to less excitation of DA neurons in the VTA and less DA release in the PFC.

Benzodiazepines

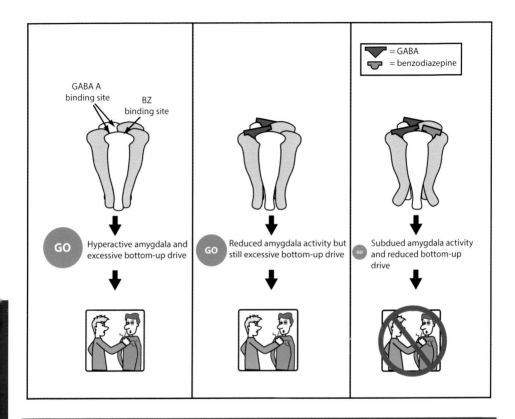

FIGURE 3.28. As modulators of GABAergic neurotransmission, benzodiazepines may help alleviate impulsively aggressive behavior. Benzodiazepines potentiate the inhibitory effects of GABA in hyperactive limbic regions, including the amygdala. Although there are data to support the use of benzodiazepines in the treatment of aggression, there are also data suggesting that benzodiazepines may actually increase aggression in some patients. In fact, whereas high doses of benzodiazepines decrease aggressive behavior, low doses have been shown to increase the number of aggressive acts. Benzodiazepines are not recommended for the long-term treatment of aggression due to their potential for addiction as well as withdrawal characterized by agitation and aggression. However, in patients with aggression and agitation due to alcohol or sedative withdrawal, the acute use of benzodiazepines may be preferred due to antipsychotics' tendency to lower the seizure threshold.

The Nonpharmacological Treatment of Aggression

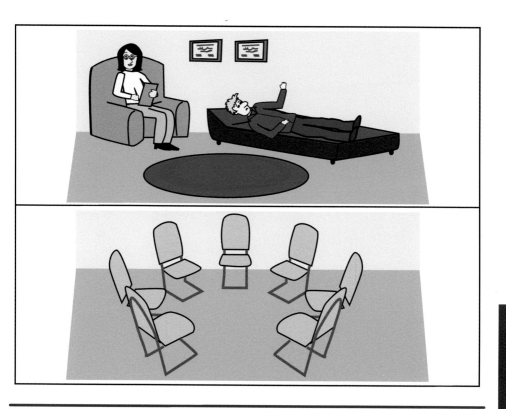

FIGURE 3.29. A combination of pharmacological and nonpharmacological treatments may be the most effective treatment for aggression. Psychosocial interventions typically work by increasing the strength of cortical top-down control. The type of psychotherapy employed should be based on the type of aggression being displayed (impulsive, psychotic, or psychopathic). For instance, anger management-based techniques may be effective for impulsive aggression but are less likely to treat psychopathic aggression (Quanbeck, 2006). Other interventions, including interpersonal skills training and structured individual counseling, have also shown effectiveness in treating impulsive aggression. Cognitive skills training may be effective in countering some of the cognitive deficits seen in many patients with psychotic aggression. Dialectical behavioral therapy, which typically takes place in a group setting, has also shown some effectiveness in reducing aggression and impulsivity (Shelton et al., 2011). Cognitive behavioral therapy has shown some degree of effectiveness in treating all 3 types of aggression, although there is very limited evidence for any treatment strategy in the case of psychopathic aggression.

- Violence can be impulsive, psychotic, or psychopathic.
- There is a high association of violence with genetic susceptibility plus an unfavorable environment.
- There are many routes to violence (e.g., mental illnesses and unfavorable factors such as substance abuse).
- Various areas of the prefrontal cortex and the amygdala are hypothetically linked to symptoms of psychotic, impulsive, and psychopathic violence.
- Understanding the topographical distribution of symptoms and their regulation by neurotransmitters provides a rationale for the psychopharmacological treatment of violence and aggression.
- There are several treatment options available for reducing the occurrence of violent or aggressive behavior; however, much of the evidence is practice-based because violent individuals are often excluded from clinical drug trials.
- Treatment with antipsychotics, especially at high doses, may be one of the most effective strategies for treating patients who are violent or aggressive.
- Although standard doses of all antipsychotics target 60-80% occupancy of D2 receptors, this may not be sufficient to quell violence and aggression in all patients.
- Pharmacokinetic treatment failure occurs when D2 receptors are inadequately occupied; such failure may be managed by high dosing, novel routes of administration, or the administration of some antipsychotics with food.
- Pharmacodynamic treatment failure occurs when patients do not respond despite achieving 80% D2 receptor occupancy; such failure can be managed by high dosing, very long treatment duration, or polypharmacy.

- Clozapine, polypharmacy, or high-dose antipsychotic monotherapy may be justified in some cases, especially if effective in reducing assaults and if side effects are carefully monitored.

- Additional strategies for managing violent or aggressive behavior include mood stabilizers, antidepressants, stimulants, adrenergic blockers, opiate antagonists, and benzodiazepines; however, evidence for the efficacy of these agents is limited and controversial.

- The addition of psychotherapy to pharmacological treatment may provide the most effective means for preventing violent or aggressive behavior.

Stahl's Illustrated | Suggested Reading

Abderhalden C, Needham I, Dassen T, et al. Predicting inpatient violence using an extended version of the Brøset-Violence-Checklist: instrument development and clinical application. BMC Psychiatry 2006;6:17.

Almvik R, Woods P. Predicting inpatient violence using the Brøset Violence Checklist (BVC). Int J Psychiatr Nurs Res 1999;4:498-505.

Anderson A, West SG. Violence against mental health professionals: when the treater becomes the victim. Innovations Clin Neurosci 2011;8:34-9.

Angelopoulou R, Lavranos G, Manolakou P. Establishing sexual dimorphism in humans. Collegium Antropologicum 2006;30:653-8.

Arato M, Frecska E, Beck C, et al. Digit length pattern in schizophrenia suggests disturbed prenatal hemispheric lateralization. Prog Neuro-Psychopharmacol Biol Psychiatry 2004;28:191-4.

Ascher-Svanum H, Faries DE, Zhu B, et al. Medication adherence and long-term functional outcomes in the treatment of schizophrenia in usual care. J Clin Psychiatry 2006;67:453-60.

Ascher-Svanum H, Nyhuis AW, Faries DE, et al. Involvement in the US criminal justice system and cost implications for persons treated for schizophrenia. BMC Psychiatry 2010;10:11.

Aslund C, Nordquist N, Comasco E, et al. Maltreatment, MAOA, and delinquency: sex differences in gene-environment interaction in a large population-based cohort of adolescents. Behav Genetics 2011;41:262-72.

Ballester J, Goldstein T, Goldstein B, et al. Is bipolar disorder specifically associated with aggression? Bipolar Disord 2012;14:283-90.

Barkataki I, Kumari V, Das M, et al. A neuropsychological investigation into violence and mental illness. Schizophr Res 2005;74:1-13.

Barkataki I, Kumari V, Das M, et al. Neural correlates of deficient response inhibition in mentally disordered violent individuals. Behav Sci Law 2008;26:51-64.

Barnes TR, Paton C. Antipsychotic polypharmacy in schizophrenia: benefits and risks. CNS Drugs 2011;25:383-99.

Barr RS, Culhane MA, Jubelt LE, et al. The effects of transdermal nicotine on cognition in nonsmokers with schizophrenia and nonpsychiatric controls. Neuropsychopharmacology 2008;33:480-90.

Bayle FJ, Leroy S, Gourion D, et al. 5HTTLPR polymorphism in schizophrenic patients: further support for association with violent suicide attempts. Am J Med Genetics B Neuropsychiatr Genetics 2003;119B:13-7.

Bevilacqua L, Carli V, Sarchiapone M, et al. Interaction between FKBP5 and childhood trauma and risk of aggressive behavior. Arch Gen Psychiatry 2012;69:62-70.

Bigelow DA, Cutler DL, Moore LJ, et al. Characteristics of state hospital patients who are hard to place. Hosp Community Psychiatry 1988;39:181-5.

Blair RJR. The neurobiology of psychopathic traits in youth. Nat Rev Neurosci 2013;14:786-99.

Bobes J, Fillat O, Arango C. Violence among schizophrenia out-patients compliant with medication: prevalence and associated factors. Acta Psychiatrica Scandinavica 2009;119:218-25.

Bourget D, Labelle A. Managing pathologic aggression in people with psychotic disorders. J Psychiatry Neurosci 2012;37:E3-4.

Brooks JH, Reddon JR. Serum testosterone in violent and nonviolent young offenders. J Clin Psychol 1996;52:475-83.

Buckley P, Citrome L, Nichita C, et al. Psychopharmacology of aggression in schizophrenia. Schizophr Bull 2011;37:930-6.

Cases O, Seif I, Grimsby J, et al. Aggressive behavior and altered amounts of brain serotonin and norepinephrine in mice lacking MAOA. Science 1995;268:1763-6.

Chengappa KN, Vasile J, Levine J, et al. Clozapine: its impact on aggressive behavior among patients in a state psychiatric hospital. Schizophr Res 2002;53:1-6.

Cicchetti D, Rogosch FA, Thibodeau EL. The effects of child maltreatment on early signs of antisocial behavior: genetic moderation by tryptophan hydroxylase, serotonin transporter, and monoamine oxidase A genes. Dev Psychopathol 2012;24:907-28.

Citrome L, Casey DE, Daniel DG, et al. Adjunctive divalproex and hostility among patients with schizophrenia receiving olanzapine or risperidone. Psychiatr Serv 2004;55(3):290-4.

Citrome L, Shope CB, Nolan KA, et al. Risperidone alone versus risperidone plus valproate in the treatment of patients with schizophrenia and hostility. Int Clin Psychopharmacol 2007;22:356-62.

Citrome L, Volavka J. Pharmacological management of acute and persistent aggression in forensic psychiatry settings. CNS Drugs 2011;25:1009-21.

Coccaro EF. Intermittent explosive disorder as a disorder of impulsive aggression for DSM-5. Am J Psychiatry 2012;169:577-88.

Coccaro EF, McCloskey MS, Fitzgerald DA, et al. Amygdala and orbitofrontal reactivity to social threat in individuals with impulsive aggression. Biol Psychiatry 2007;62:168-78.

Coccaro EF, Sripada CS, Yanowitch RN, et al. Corticolimbic function in impulsive aggressive behavior. Biol Psychiatry 2011;69:1153-9.

Collinson SL, Lim M, Chaw JH, et al. Increased ratio of 2nd to 4th digit (2D:4D) in schizophrenia. Psychiatry Res 2010;176:8-12.

Comai S, Tau M, Gobbi G. The psychopharmacology of aggressive behavior: a translational approach: part 1: neurobiology. J Clin Psychopharmacol 2012a;32:83-94.

Comai S, Tau M, Pavlovic Z, et al. The psychopharmacology of aggressive behavior: a translational approach: part 2: clinical studies using atypical antipsychotics, anticonvulsants, and lithium. J Clin Psychopharmacol 2012b;32:237-60.

Correll CU. From receptor pharmacology to improved outcomes: individualising the selection, dosing, and switching of antipsychotics. Eur Psychiatry 2010;25(suppl 2):S12-21.

Correll CU, Rummel-Kluge C, Corves C, et al. Antipsychotic combinations vs monotherapy in schizophrenia: a meta-analysis of randomized controlled trials. Schizophr Bull 2009;35:443-57.

Davis JM, Chen N. Dose response and dose equivalence of antipsychotics. J Clin Psychopharmacol 2004;24:192-208.

De Sanctis P, Foxe JJ, Czobor P, et al. Early sensory-perceptual processing deficits for affectively valenced inputs are more pronounced in schizophrenia patients with a history of violence than in their nonviolent peers. Soc Cognitive Affective Neurosci 2013;8(6):678-87.

Dean K, Walsh E, Moran P, et al. Violence in women with psychosis in the community: prospective study. Br J Psychiatry 2006;188:264-70.

Denson TF, Ronay R, von Hippel W, et al. Endogenous testosterone and cortisol modulate neural responses during induced anger control. Soc Neurosci 2013;8:165-77.

Dussias P, Kalali AH, Citrome L. Polypharmacy of schizophrenia. Psychiatry (Edgmont) 2010;7:17-9.

Essock SM, Schooler NR, Stroup TS, et al. Effectiveness of switching from antipsychotic polypharmacy to monotherapy. Am J Psychiatry 2011;168:702-8.

Faries D, Ascher-Svanum H, Zhu B, et al. Antipsychotic monotherapy and polypharmacy in the naturalistic treatment of schizophrenia with atypical antipsychotics. BMC Psychiatry 2005;5:26.

Fazel S, Grann M. The population impact of severe mental illness on violent crime. Am J Psychiatry 2006;163:1397-403.

Fazel S, Grann M, Carlstrom E, et al. Risk factors for violent crime in schizophrenia: a national cohort study of 13,806 patients. J Clin Psychiatry 2009a;70:362-9.

Fazel S, Gulati G, Linsell L, et al. Schizophrenia and violence: systematic review and meta-analysis. PLOS Med 2009b;6:e1000120.

Fazel S, Langstrom N, Hjern A, et al. Schizophrenia, substance abuse, and violent crime. JAMA 2009c;301:2016-23.

Fazel S, Lichtenstein P, Grann M, et al. Bipolar disorder and violent crime: new evidence from population-based longitudinal studies and systematic review. Arch Gen Psychiatry 2010;67:931-8.

Fazel S, Singh JP, Doll H, et al. Use of risk assessment instruments to predict violence and antisocial behaviour in 73 samples involving 24 827 people: systematic review and meta-analysis. BMJ 2012;345:e4692.

Fergusson DM, Boden JM, Horwood LJ, et al. MAOA, abuse exposure and antisocial behaviour: 30-year longitudinal study. Br J Psychiatry 2011;198:457-63.

Flannery RB Jr. Repetitively assaultive psychiatric patients: review of published findings, 1978-2001. Psychiatr Q 2002;73:229-37.

Frogley C, Taylor D, Dickens G, et al. A systematic review of the evidence of clozapine's antiaggressive effects. Int J Neuropsychopharmacol 2012;15:1351-71.

Gillies D, Sampson S, Beck A, et al. Benzodiazepines for psychosis-induced aggression or agitation. Cochrane Database Syst Rev 2013;4:CD003079.

Glenn AL, Johnson AK, Raine A. Antisocial personality disorder: a current review. Curr Psychiatry Rep 2013;15(12):427.

Glenn AL, Raine A. The neurobiology of psychopathy. Psychiatr Clin North Am 2008;31:463-75, vii.

Goldstein JM, Seidman LJ, Makris N, et al. Hypothalamic abnormalities in schizophrenia: sex effects and genetic vulnerability. Biol Psychiatry 2007;61:935-45.

Goldstein JM, Seidman LJ, O'Brien LM, et al. Impact of normal sexual dimorphisms on sex differences in structural brain abnormalities in schizophrenia assessed by magnetic resonance imaging. Arch Gen Psychiatry 2002;59:154-64.

Gray NS, Hill C, McGleish A, et al. Prediction of violence and self-harm in mentally disordered offenders: a prospective study of the efficacy of HCR-20, PCL-R, and psychiatric symptomatology. J Consult Clin Psychol 2003;71:443-51.

Green MF, Kern RS, Heaton RK. Longitudinal studies of cognition and functional outcome in schizophrenia: implications for MATRICS. Schizophr Res 2004;72:41-51.

Greenfield TK, McNiel DE, Binder RL. Violent behavior and length of psychiatric hospitalization. Hosp Community Psychiatry 1989;40:809-14.

Gregory S, Ffytche D, Simmons A, et al. The antisocial brain: psychopathy matters. Arch Gen Psychiatry 2012;69(9):962-72.

Guillem F, Mendrek A, Lavoie ME, et al. Sex differences in memory processing in schizophrenia: an event-related potential (ERP) study. Prog Neuropsychopharmacol Biol Psychiatry 2009;33:1-10.

Gur RE, Kohler C, Turetsky BI, et al. A sexually dimorphic ratio of orbitofrontal to amygdala volume is altered in schizophrenia. Biol Psychiatry 2004;55:512-7.

Guy LS, Douglas KS. Examining the utility of the PCL:SV as a screening measure using competing factor models of psychopathy. Psychol Assess 2006;18:225-30.

Haller J. The neurobiology of abnormal manifestations of aggression—a review of hypothalamic mechanisms in cats, rodents, and humans. Brain Res Bull 2013;93:97-109.

Han DH, Kee BS, Min KJ, et al. Effects of catechol-O-methyltransferase Val158Met polymorphism on the cognitive stability and aggression in the first-onset schizophrenic patients. Neuroreport 2006;17(1):95-9.

Hare RD, Neumann CS. Psychopathy as a clinical and empirical construct. Annu Rev Clin Psychol 2008;4:217-46.

Herings RM, Erkens JA. Increased suicide attempt rate among patients interrupting use of atypical antipsychotics. Pharmacoepidemiol Drug Safety 2003;12:423-4.

Herrera JN, Sramek JJ, Costa JF, et al. High potency neuroleptics and violence in schizophrenics. J Nerv Ment Dis 1988;176:558-61.

Holden C. Sex and the suffering brain. Science 2005;308:1574.

Hoptman MJ, Antonius D. Neuroimaging correlates of aggression in schizophrenia: an update. Curr Opinion Psychiatry 2011;24:100-6.

Huber TJ, Tettenborn C, Leifke E, et al. Sex hormones in psychotic men. Psychoneuroendocrinology 2005;30:111-4.

Ikai S, Remington G, Suzuki T, et al. A cross-sectional study of plasma risperidone levels with risperidone long-acting injectable: implications for dopamine D2 receptor occupancy during maintenance treatment in schizophrenia. J Clin Psychiatry 2012;73:1147-52.

Kane JM. The use of higher-dose antipsychotic medication. Comment on the Royal College of Psychiatrists' consensus statement. Br J Psychiatry 1994;164:431-2.

Kim JJ, Shih JC, Chen K, et al. Selective enhancement of emotional, but not motor, learning in monoamine oxidase A-deficient mice. Proc Natl Acad Sci U S A 1997;94:5929-33.

Ko YH, Jung SW, Joe SH, et al. Association between serum testosterone levels and the severity of negative symptoms in male patients with chronic schizophrenia. Psychoneuroendocrinology 2007;32:385-91.

Konarzewska B, Wolczynski S, Szulc A, et al. Effect of risperidone and olanzapine on reproductive hormones, psychopathology and sexual functioning in male patients with schizophrenia. Psychoneuroendocrinology 2009;34:129-39.

Kosson DS, Lorenz AR, Newman JP. Effects of comorbid psychopathy on criminal offending and emotion processing in male offenders with antisocial personality disorder. J Abnorm Psychol 2006;115(4):798-806.

Kotler M, Barak P, Cohen H, et al. Homicidal behavior in schizophrenia associated with a genetic polymorphism determining low catechol-O-methyltransferase (COMT) activity. Am J Med Genetics 1999;88:628-33.

Krakowski MI, Convit A, Jaeger J, et al. Neurological impairment in violent schizophrenic inpatients. Am J Psychiatry 1989;146:849-53.

Krakowski MI, Czobor P. Executive function predicts response to antiaggression treatment in schizophrenia: a randomized controlled trial. J Clin Psychiatry 2012;73:74-80.

Krakowski MI, Czobor P, Citrome L, et al. Atypical antipsychotic agents in the treatment of violent patients with schizophrenia and schizoaffective disorder. Arch Gen Psychiatry 2006;63:622-9.

Krakowski MI, Czobor P, Nolan KA. Atypical antipsychotics, neurocognitive deficits, and aggression in schizophrenic patients. J Clin Psychopharmacol 2008;28(5):485-93.

Krakowski MI, Kunz M, Czobor P, et al. Long-term high-dose neuroleptic treatment: who gets it and why? Hosp Community Psychiatry 1993;44:640-4.

Kumari V, Aasen I, Taylor P, et al. Neural dysfunction and violence in schizophrenia: an fMRI investigation. Schizophr Res 2006;84:144-64.

Kumari V, Barkataki I, Goswami S, et al. Dysfunctional, but not functional, impulsivity is associated with a history of seriously violent behaviour and reduced orbitofrontal and hippocampal volumes in schizophrenia. Psychiatry Res 2009;173:39-44.

Lachman HM, Nolan KA, Mohr P, et al. Association between catechol-O-methyltransferase genotype and violence in schizophrenia and schizoaffective disorder. Am J Psychiatry 1998;155:835-7.

Langle G, Steinert T, Weiser P, et al. Effects of polypharmacy on outcome in patients with schizophrenia in routine psychiatric treatment. Acta Psychiatrica Scandinavica 2012;125:372-81.

Large MM, Nielssen O. Violence in first-episode psychosis: a systematic review and meta-analysis. Schizophr Res 2011;125:209-20.

Lavranos G, Angelopoulou R, Manolakou P, et al. Hormonal and meta-hormonal determinants of sexual dimorphism. Collegium Antropologicum 2006;30:659-63.

Lee AMR, Galynker II. Violence in bipolar disorder: what role does childhood trauma play? Psychiatr Times 2010;27:32-4.

Lidz CW, Mulvey EP, Gardner W. The accuracy of predictions of violence to others. JAMA 1993;269:1007-11.

Lindenmayer JP, Liu-Seifert H, Kulkarni PM, et al. Medication nonadherence and treatment outcome in patients with schizophrenia or schizoaffective disorder with suboptimal prior response. J Clin Psychiatry 2009;70:990-6.

Maghsoodloo S, Ghodousi A, Karimzadeh T. The relationship of antisocial personality disorder and history of conduct disorder with crime incidence in schizophrenia. J Res Med Sci 2012;17(6):566-71.

Manning JT, Scutt D, Wilson J, et al. The ratio of 2nd to 4th digit length: a predictor of sperm numbers and concentrations of testosterone, luteinizing hormone and oestrogen. Hum Reprod 1998;13:3000-4.

Manuck SB, Flory JD, Ferrell RE, et al. Aggression and anger-related traits associated with a polymorphism of the tryptophan hydroxylase gene. Biol Psychiatry 1999;45:603-14.

Marder SR. Overview of partial compliance. J Clin Psychiatry 2003;64(suppl 16):3-9.

Mattes JA. Medications for aggressiveness in prison: focus on oxcarbazepine. J Am Acad Psychiatry Law 2012;40:234-8.

Mauri MC, Volonteri LS, Colasanti A, et al. Clinical pharmacokinetics of atypical antipsychotics: a critical review of the relationship between plasma concentrations and clinical response. Clin Pharmacokinet 2007;46:359-88.

McDermott R, Tingley D, Cowden J, et al. Monoamine oxidase A gene (MAOA) predicts behavioral aggression following provocation. Proc Natl Acad Sci U S A 2009;106:2118-23.

McGuire J. A review of effective interventions for reducing aggression and violence. Philos Trans Royal Soc B Biol Sci 2008;363:2577-97.

McIntyre MH. The use of digit ratios as markers for perinatal androgen action. Reprod Biol Endocrinol 2006;4:10.

Mendrek A, Stip E. Sexual dimorphism in schizophrenia: is there a need for gender-based protocols? Expert Rev Neurother 2011;11:951-9.

Meyer-Lindenberg A, Buckholtz JW, Kolachana B, et al. Neural mechanisms of genetic risk of impulsivity and violence in humans. Proc Natl Acad Sci U S A 2006;103:6269-74.

Meyers B, D'Agostino A, Walker J, et al. Gonadectomy and hormone replacement exert region- and enzyme isoform-specific effects on monoamine oxidase and catechol-O-methyltransferase activity in prefrontal cortex and neostriatum of adult male rats. Neuroscience 2010;165:850-62.

Milev P, Ho BC, Arndt S, et al. Predictive values of neurocognition and negative symptoms on functional outcome in schizophrenia: a longitudinal first-episode study with 7-year follow-up. Am J Psychiatry 2005;162:495-506.

Moore L, Kyaw M, Vercammen A, et al. Serum testosterone levels are related to cognitive function in men with schizophrenia. Psychoneuroendocrinology 2013;38:1717-28.

Morgan CP, Bale TL. Early prenatal stress epigenetically programs dysmasculinization in second-generation offspring via the paternal lineage. J Neurosci 2011;31:11748-55.

Morrissette DA, Stahl SM. Optimizing outcomes in schizophrenia: long-acting depots and long-term treatment. CNS Spectrums 2012;17:(suppl 1):10-21.

National Institutes of Mental Health Psychoactive Drug Screening Program. Web site. http://pdsp.med.unc.edu/indexR.html. Accessed Feb 1, 2013.

Nikisch G, Baumann P, Kiessling B, et al. Relationship between dopamine D2 receptor occupancy, clinical response, and drug and monoamine metabolites levels in plasma and cerebrospinal fluid. A pilot study in patients suffering from first-episode schizophrenia treated with quetiapine. J Psychiatr Res 2010;44:754-9.

Nolan KA, Czobor P, Roy BB, et al. Characteristics of assaultive behavior among psychiatric inpatients. Psychiatr Serv 2003;54:1012-6.

Nord M, Farde L. Antipsychotic occupancy of dopamine receptors in schizophrenia. CNS Neurosci Ther 2011;17:97-103.

Ohmura Y, Tsutsui-Kimura I, Yoshioka M. Impulsive behavior and nicotinic acetylcholine receptors. J Pharmacol Sci 2012;118:413-22.

Oliver-Africano P, Murphy D, Tyrer P. Aggressive behaviour in adults with intellectual disability: defining the role of drug treatment. CNS Drugs 2009;23:903-13.

Paus T, Otaky N, Caramanos Z, et al. In vivo morphometry of the intrasulcal gray matter in the human cingulate, paracingulate, and superior-rostral sulci: hemispheric asymmetries, gender differences and probability maps. J Comp Neurol 1996;376:664-73.

Pavlov KA, Chistiakov DA, Chekhonin VP. Genetic determinants of aggression and impulsivity in humans. J Appl Genetics 2012;53:61-82.

Quanbeck C. Forensic psychiatric aspects of inpatient violence. Psychiatr Clin North Am 2006;29:743-60.

Quanbeck CD, McDermott BE, Lam J, et al. Categorization of aggressive acts committed by chronically assaultive state hospital patients. Psychiatr Serv 2007;58:521-8.

Rasanen P, Hakko H, Visuri S, et al. Serum testosterone levels, mental disorders and criminal behaviour. Acta Psychiatrica Scandinavica 1999;99:348-52.

Remington G, Kapur S. Antipsychotic dosing: how much but also how often? Schizophr Bull 2010;36:900-3.

Retz W, Retz-Junginger P, Supprian T, et al. Association of serotonin transporter promoter gene polymorphism with violence: relation with personality disorders, impulsivity, and childhood ADHD psychopathology. Behav Sci Law 2004;22:415-25.

Robb AS, Carson WH, Nyilas M, et al. Changes in positive and negative syndrome scale-derived hostility factor in adolescents with schizophrenia treated with aripiprazole: post hoc analysis of randomized clinical trial data. J Child Adolesc Psychopharmacol 2010;20:33-8.

Rosell DR, Thompson JL, Slifstein M, et al. Increased serotonin 2A receptor availability in the orbitofrontal cortex of physically aggressive personality disordered patients. Biol Psychiatry 2010;67:1154-62.

Rothemund Y, Zeigler S, Hermann C, et al. Fear conditioning in psychopaths: event-related potentials and peripheral measures. Biol Psychol 2012;90(1):50-9.

Schwartz TL, Stahl SM. Treatment strategies for dosing the second generation antipsychotics. CNS Neurosci Ther 2011;17:110-7.

Seeman P. Dopamine D2 receptors as treatment targets in schizophrenia. Clin Schizophr Related Psychoses 2010;4:56-73.

Serper M, Beech DR, Harvey PD, et al. Neuropsychological and symptom predictors of aggression on the psychiatric inpatient service. J Clin Exp Neuropsychol 2008;30:700-9.

Shelton D, Kesten K, Zhang W, et al. Impact of dialectic behavior therapy-corrections modified (DBT-CM) upon behaviorally challenged incarcerated male adolescents. J Child Adolesc Psychiatr Nurs 2011;24(2):105-13.

Shrivastava A, Shah N, Johnston M, et al. Predictors of long-term outcome of first-episode schizophrenia: a ten-year follow-up study. Indian J Psychiatry 2010;52:320-6.

Siever LJ. Neurobiology of aggression and violence. Am J Psychiatry 2008;165:429-42.

Singh JP, Grann M, Fazel S. A comparative study of violence risk assessment tools: a systematic review and metaregression analysis of 68 studies involving 25,980 participants. Clin Psychol Rev 2011a;31:499-513.

Singh JP, Grann M, Lichtenstein P, et al. A novel approach to determining violence risk in schizophrenia: developing a stepped strategy in 13,806 discharged patients. PLOS ONE 2012a;7:e31727.

Singh JP, Serper M, Reinharth J, et al. Structured assessment of violence risk in schizophrenia and other psychiatric disorders: a systematic review of the validity, reliability, and item content of 10 available instruments. Schizophr Bull 2011b;37:899-912.

Singh JP, Volavka J, Czobor P, et al. A meta-analysis of the Val158Met COMT polymorphism and violent behavior in schizophrenia. PLOS ONE 2012b;7:e43423.

Sjoberg RL, Ducci F, Barr CS, et al. A non-additive interaction of a functional MAO-A VNTR and testosterone predicts antisocial behavior. Neuropsychopharmacology 2008;33:425-30.

Skeem JL, Manchak SM, Lidz CW, et al. The utility of patients' self-perceptions of violence risk: consider asking the person who may know best. Psychiatr Serv 2013;64:410-5.

Snyder MA, Gao WJ. NMDA hypofunction as a convergence point for progression and symptoms of schizophrenia. Frontiers Cell Neurosci 2013;7:31.

Song H, Min SK. Aggressive behavior model in schizophrenic patients. Psychiatry Res 2009;167:58-65.

Soyka M. Neurobiology of aggression and violence in schizophrenia. Schizophr Bull 2011;37:913-20.

Stahl SM. Antipsychotic polypharmacy: never say never, but never say always. Acta Psychiatrica Scandinavica 2012;125:349-51.

Stahl SM. Stahl's essential psychopharmacology: neuroscientific basis and practical applications. 4th ed. New York, NY: Cambridge University Press; 2013.

Stahl SM. Stahl's essential psychopharmacology: the prescriber's guide. 4th ed. New York, NY: Cambridge University Press; 2011.

Stahl SM, Grady MM. A critical review of atypical antipsychotic utilization: comparing monotherapy with polypharmacy and augmentation. Curr Med Chem 2004;11:313-27.

Stilwell EN, Yates SE, Brahm NC. Violence among persons diagnosed with schizophrenia: how pharmacists can help. Res Soc Adm Pharm 2011;7:421-9.

Suzuki T, Uchida H, Tanaka KF, et al. Revising polypharmacy to a single antipsychotic regimen for patients with chronic schizophrenia. Int J Neuropsychopharmacol 2004;7:133-42.

Swanson JW, Swartz MS, Van Dorn RA, et al. Comparison of antipsychotic medication effects on reducing violence in people with schizophrenia. Br J Psychiatry 2008;193:37-43.

Taherianfard M, Shariaty M. Evaluation of serum steroid hormones in schizophrenic patients. Indian J Med Sci 2004;58:3-9.

Takahashi T, Suzuki M, Kawasaki Y, et al. Perigenual cingulate gyrus volume in patients with schizophrenia: a magnetic resonance imaging study. Biol Psychiatry 2003;53:593-600.

Tauscher J, Kapur S. Choosing the right dose of antipsychotics in schizophrenia: lessons from neuroimaging studies. CNS Drugs 2001;15:671-8.

Taylor DM, Smith L, Gee SH, et al. Augmentation of clozapine with a second antipsychotic—a meta-analysis. Acta Psychiatrica Scandinavica 2012;125:15-24.

Taylor PJ, Bragado-Jimenez MD. Women, psychosis and violence. Int J Law Psychiatry 2009;32:56-64.

Teo AR, Holley SR, Leary M, et al. The relationship between level of training and accuracy of violence risk assessment. Psychiatr Serv 2012;63:1089-94.

Thompson C. The use of high-dose antipsychotic medication. Br J Psychiatry 1994;164:448-58.

Thompson JM, Sonuga-Barke EJ, Morgan AR, et al. The catechol-O-methyltransferase (COMT) Val158Met polymorphism moderates the effect of antenatal stress on childhood behavioural problems: longitudinal evidence across multiple ages. Dev Med Child Neurol 2012;54:148-54.

Tolman AO, Mullendore KB. Risk evaluations for the courts: is service quality a function of specialization? Professional Psychol Res Pract 2003;34:225-32.

Topiwala A, Fazel S. The pharmacological management of violence in schizophrenia: a structured review. Expert Rev Neurother 2011;11:53-63.

Uchida H, Takeuchi H, Graff-Guerrero A, et al. Predicting dopamine D2 receptor occupancy from plasma levels of antipsychotic drugs: a systematic review and pooled analysis. J Clin Psychopharmacol 2011;31:318-25.

Volavka J, Citrome L. Heterogeneity of violence in schizophrenia and implications for long-term treatment. Int J Clin Pract 2008;62:1237-45.

Volavka J, Citrome LL. Psychopharmacology of aggression and violence in mental illness: a review of evidence-based treatments. Psychiatr Times 2012;29(4):26-33.

Volavka J, Czobor P, Nolan K, et al. Overt aggression and psychotic symptoms in patients with schizophrenia treated with clozapine, olanzapine, risperidone, or haloperidol. J Clin Psychopharmacol 2004;24:225-8.

Volman I, Toni I, Verhagen L, et al. Endogenous testosterone modulates prefrontal-amygdala connectivity during social emotional behavior. Cereb Cortex 2011;21:2282-90.

Wehring HJ, Carpenter WT. Violence and schizophrenia. Schizophr Bull 2011;37:877-8.

Weiden PJ, Kozma C, Grogg A, et al. Partial compliance and risk of rehospitalization among California Medicaid patients with schizophrenia. Psychiatr Serv 2004;55:886-91.

Wilkie A, Preston N, Wesby R. High dose neuroleptics—who gives them and why? Psychiatr Bull 2001;25:179-83.

Winstanley CA, Theobald DE, Dalley JW, et al. 5-HT2A and 5-HT2C receptor antagonists have opposing effects on a measure of impulsivity: interactions with global 5-HT depletion. Psychopharmacology (Berl) 2004;176:376-85.

Wu JB, Chen K, Li Y, et al. Regulation of monoamine oxidase A by the SRY gene on the Y chromosome. FASEB J 2009;23:4029-38.

Yang M, Wong SC, Coid J. The efficacy of violence prediction: a meta-analytic comparison of nine risk assessment tools. Psychol Bull 2010;136:740-67.

Zammit S, Jones G, Jones SJ, et al. Polymorphisms in the MAOA, MAOB, and COMT genes and aggressive behavior in schizophrenia. Am J Med Genetics B Neuropsychiatr Genetics 2004;128B:19-20.

benzodiazepines 78
bipolar disorder
  and substance abuse 8
  and violent behavior 19
borderline personality disorder 28
bottom-up limbic drive 25, 27
  suppression of 50
Brøset Violence Checklist (BVC) 21

carbamazepine 73
catechol-O-methyltransferase see COMT
child abuse
  MAO-A gene 44
  and violence 7
citalopram 74
Classification of Violence Risk (COVR) 21
Clinically Feasible Iterative Classification Tree
      (ICT-CF) 21
clozapine
  binding profile 58
  dose range 71
  high-dose monotherapy 61
cognitive behavioral therapy 79
cognitive dysfunction 18
  testosterone-induced 16
command hallucinations 4
COMT 46, 48
conduct disorder 31
cortical control centers 25, 26
counseling 79

delusions 4
dialectical behavioral therapy 79
dopamine 35
  and aggression 36
  D2 receptor occupancy 52, 60
dose ranges of atypical antipsychotics 71

emotional hypersensitivity 3

FKBP5 48
fluoxetine 74

GABA see gamma-aminobutyric acid
gamma-aminobutyric acid (GABA) 35
  and aggression 39

gender
  sexual dimorphism
    MAO-A gene 44
    reversal in schizophrenia 12
    and testosterone exposure 13
  "sexual unmorphism" 12
  and violence 11
genes associated with aggression
    5HTTLPR 47, 48
    COMT 46, 48
    FKBP5 48
    MAO-A see MAO-A gene
genetics of aggression 23
glutamate 35
  and aggression 39
grandiosity 4
gray matter, reduced volume 33

Hare Psychopathy Checklist: Screening Version
      (PCL:SV) 21
Hare Psychopathy Checklist–Revised (PCL-R) 21
heterogeneity of violence 2
high-dose monotherapy
    atypical antipsychotics 61–71
    conventional antipsychotics 72
hippocampus 27
Historical Clinical Risk Management (HCR-20) 21
hostility, testosterone-induced 16
5HTTLPR 47, 48
hypothalamic–pituitary–adrenal (HPA) axis 7
hypothalamus 27

iloperidone
  binding profile 58
  dose range 71
  high-dose monotherapy 68
impulsive aggression 2, 3
    MAO-A gene 45
    neurocircuitry 28
    and serotonin 15
    and testosterone 15
inheritance of aggression 41
interpersonal skills training 79

lamotrigine 73
limbic control centers 25, 27

lithium 73
lurasidone
  binding profile 58
  dose range 71
  high-dose monotherapy 70

MAO-A gene 42, 48
  child abuse 44
  polymorphisms, and impulsivity 45
  sexual dimorphism 44
  testosterone regulation 43
men
  childhood abuse 44
  schizophrenia in 12
  violent behavior 11
Modified Screening Tool (MST) 21
monoamine oxidase A ("warrior gene")
        see MAO-A gene
mood stabilizers 73
  see also individual drugs

naltrexone 77
neurobiology 23
  aggression 24
    impulsive 29
    neurotransmitter systems 35
    psychopathic 32
    psychotic 29
  bottom-up limbic drive 25, 27
  impaired neurotransmission 24
  testosterone effects 17
  top-down cortical brake 25, 26
nonpharmacological treatment 79
norepinephrine 35
nucleus accumbens 29

olanzapine
  binding profile 58
  dose range 71
  high-dose monotherapy 62
opiate antagonists 77
orbitofrontal cortex 26
oxcarbazepine 73

paliperidone
  binding profile 58

dose range 71
  high-dose monotherapy 64
paranoid 4
phenytoin 73
posttraumatic stress disorder (PTSD) 28
predatory gain 5
prediction of violence 22
prefrontal cortex 26, 35
psychopathic aggression 2, 5
  neurocircuitry 32
Psychopathology Checklist–Revised (PCL-R) 30
psychopathy 30
  antisocial personality disorder 31
  conduct disorder 31
  reduced gray matter volume 33
psychosis 4
psychosocial interventions 79
psychotic aggression 2, 4
  neurocircuitry 29

quetiapine
  binding profile 58
  dose range 71
  high-dose monotherapy 65

reactive aggression 2, 3
remorse, lack of 5
risk assessment 21, 22
risk factors for violence 6
  affective disorder 19
  child abuse 7
  cognitive dysfunction 18
  gender 11
  schizophrenia 9, 10
  substance abuse 8
  treatment nonadherence 20
risperidone
  binding profile 58
  dose range 71
  high-dose monotherapy 63

schizophrenia
  delusions 4
  "sexual unmorphism" 12
  and substance abuse 8

CME: Posttest and Certificate

Release/Expiration Dates

Released: March 1, 2014

CME Credit Expires: February 28, 2017. *If this date has passed, please contact NEI for updated information.*

CME Posttest Study Guide

PLEASE NOTE: The posttest can only be submitted online. The posttest questions have been provided below solely as a study tool to help prepare you for your online submission. ***Faxed/ mailed copies of the posttest cannot be processed*** *and will be returned to the sender. If you do not have access to the Internet, contact NEI customer service at 888-535-5600.*

1. Jill is a 33-year-old patient who was recently arrested for assaulting her father with a sledgehammer. The assault was instigated by the patient's hallucination that her father had crickets all over his face, indicating only partial response to her current clozapine treatment. What are potential evidence-based treatment strategies for psychotic patients with inadequate response to clozapine?

   A. Raise clozapine dose to 1200 mg/day

   B. Switch to aripiprazole 45 mg/day

   C. Augment with a second antipsychotic

   D. A and C only

   E. B and C only

2. A 46-year-old male patient with psychotic aggression is unable to take clozapine due to a history of thrombocytopenia. Which of the following is a reasonable approach to treatment-resistant psychosis when clozapine is not an option?

   A. Dose olanzapine >40 mg/day

   B. Dose quetiapine to 1800 mg/day

   C. Dose ziprasidone to 320 mg/day

   D. All of the above

   E. None of the above

3. Charles is a 32-year-old patient with schizoaffective disorder and a history of childhood abuse. Genetic testing has revealed that he is homozygous for the short (3-repeat) allele of the MAO-A gene. Compared to another male patient with schizoaffective disorder and a history of child abuse who is homozygous for the long (4-repeat) allele of the MAO-A gene:

A. Charles has an increased risk of violent behavior

B. Charles has a decreased risk of violent behavior

C. The risk of violent behavior is the same for both of these male patients

4. Fred is a 29-year-old patient with untreated schizophrenia. He was recently institutionalized secondary to assaulting 4 individuals on the subway whom he believed to be aliens. With regard to dysfunctional neurocircuitry, psychotic aggression is believed to be driven by hyperactivity in which brain region?

A. Prefrontal cortex

B. Striatum

C. Amygdala

5. If olanzapine is dosed so that 60% occupancy of dopamine D2 receptors takes place, which of the following might be expected:

A. Sedation due to binding at histaminic H1 receptors

B. Cardiometabolic effects due to binding at serotonergic 5HT2C receptors

C. Cardiometabolic effects due to binding at muscarinic M3 receptors

D. Improvement in anxiety due to binding at serotonergic 5HT1A receptors

E. A and B only

F. C and D only

6. In male patients with schizophrenia, decreased testosterone is associated with:

A. An increased risk of violence and aggression

B. A decreased risk of violence and aggression

C. Neither an increased nor a decreased risk of violence and aggression

7. Individuals with psychopathic aggression have:

A. A hyperactive amygdala and a hyperactive prefrontal cortex

B. A hyperactive amygdala and a hypoactive prefrontal cortex

C. A hypoactive amygdala and a hypoactive prefrontal cortex

D. A hypoactive amygdala and a hyperactive prefrontal cortex

8. Toby is a 32-year-old male patient with bipolar disorder. He has a history of incarcerations due to acts of impulsive aggression, including a fist fight at a sporting event that left the victim hospitalized in a coma. His clinician is considering augmenting his current mood stabilizer (lamotrigine) with lithium. To decrease aggressive behavior, lithium should be dosed:

A. Higher than for the treatment of acute bipolar mania

B. Lower than for the treatment of acute bipolar mania

C. The same as for the treatment of acute bipolar mania

9. A 55-year-old patient with a history of alcohol abuse presents to emergency services in acute alcohol withdrawal and physically assaults 2 of the emergency room staff. When treating aggression using a benzodiazepine:

A. The dose administered should be relatively low

B. The dose administered should be relatively high

C. Long-term use is not recommended

D. A and C only

E. B and C only

10. Stimulants may be hypothetically effective in treating impulsive aggression because they:

A. Decrease the reuptake of norepinephrine and dopamine

B. Immediately lower norepinephrine and dopamine levels

C. Lead to down-regulation or desensitization of norepinephrine and dopamine receptors

CME Online Posttest and Certificate

To receive your certificate of CME credit or participation, complete the posttest and activity evaluation available only online at **www.neiglobal.com/CME** (under "Book"). If a passing score of 70% or more is attained (required to receive credit), you can immediately print your certificate. There is a fee for the posttest (waived for NEI members). If you have questions or do not have access to the Internet, contact customer service at 888-535-5600.

Printed in the United States
By Bookmasters